NATIONAL BOARDS EXAMINATION REVIEW

FOR PART III

NATIONAL BOARDS EXAMINATION REVIEW

FOR PART III

200 MULTIPLE-CHOICE QUESTIONS WITH EXPLANATORY ANSWERS, PLUS 15 PATIENT MANAGEMENT PROBLEMS

SECOND EDITION

Barbara Ann Allen, PhD
James R. Allen, MD
Patrick K. C. Chun, MD
William P. Coleman III, MD
Ralph W. Hale, MD
Lee Hixson, MD
Victor LaCerva, MD
John Lederer, MD
Alvin E. Parrish, MD
William Pryse-Phillips, MD
M. D. Ram, MD
William A. Sodeman, Jr, MD
Barry M. Stults, MD

MEDICAL EXAMINATION PUBLISHING COMPANY

No responsibility is assumed by the publisher for any injury and/or damage to persons or property as a matter of products liability, negligence, or otherwise, or from any use or operation of any methods, products, instructions, or ideas contained in the material herein. No suggested test or procedure should be carried out unless, in the reader's judgment, its risk is justified. Because the drugs specified within this book may not have specific approval by the Food and Drug Administration in regard to the indications and dosages that are recommended by the authors, we recommend that independent verification of diagnoses should be made. Discussions, views, and recommendations as to medical procedures, choice of drugs, and drug dosages are the responsibility of the authors.

Medical Examination Publishing Company
A Division of Elsevier Science Publishing Co., Inc.
655 Avenue of the Americas, New York, New York 10010

Library of Congress Cataloging-in-Publication Data

National boards examination review for part III.
Includes bibliographies.
1. Medicine–Examinations, questions, etc., I. Allen, Barbara Ann.
[DNLM: 1. Medicine–examination, questions. W 18 N2766]
R834.5.N38 1989 610'.76 88-34522
ISBN 0-444-01462-4

Current printing (last digit):
10 9 8 7 6 5 4

Manufactured in the United States of America

Contents

Preface vii
Contributors ix

1 **Therapy and Management** 1
Explanatory Answers 25
References 45

2 **Pictorial** 47
Explanatory Answers 97
References 118

3 **Patient Management Problems** 120
Instructions 120
Problems 122
Scoring System 181
Scoring and Discussion 182
Responses 235

Preface

This second edition of *National Boards Examination Review for Part III* offers a comprehensive review designed to determine one's ability to use medical knowledge in solving a variety of clinical problems encountered in the first year of postgraduate training. It is specifically designed to prepare the candidate for National Boards Part III.

Just like the actual examination, this book is divided into three sections. The first is composed of 100 multiple-choice questions devoted to therapy and management. The second section integrates 38 illustrations with 100 multiple-choice questions intended to help sharpen skills in interpreting graphic and pictorial material relating to the management of patients.

All questions have been modeled after those used on the Boards and are arranged by type to provide practice in dealing with various test formats. Explanatory answers and references are conveniently placed at the end of the section containing the corresponding questions.

The third section comprises 15 patient management problems covering the fields of cardiology, dermatology, gastroenterology, nephrology, neurology, obstetrics and gynecology, pediatrics, psychiatry, and surgery. These problems place the reader in the position of the clinician and offer immediate feedback from the decisions made across the continuum of patient care. Included with the problems are 27 illustrations to guide the reader in the selection of appropriate differential diagnoses.

Using this book you may identify areas of relative strength and weakness in your command of the constituent disciplines. Specific references to widely used textbooks allow you to return to authoritative sources for further study. The explanatory answers are intended to prompt thought about the choices – correct and incorrect – to put the responses in broadened perspective, and to add to your fund of knowledge. In composite, the material in this book emphasizes problem solving and the application of underlying principles, in addition to factual recall.

Contributors

Barbara Ann Allen, PhD, *Clinical Associate Professor,* Department of Psychiatry and Behavioral Sciences, University of Oklahoma, Tulsa Medical College; and *Director,* Tulsa Mental Health Council and Crisis Center, Tulsa, Oklahoma

James R. Allen, MD, FRCP(C), *Professor and Chairman,* Department of Psychiatry and Behavioral Sciences, University of Oklahoma, Tulsa Medical College; and *Director,* Tulsa Psychiatric Center, Tulsa, Oklahoma

Patrick K. C. Chun, MD, FACP, FACC, FCCP, Cardiology Service, Valley Diagnostic Clinic, Harlingen, Texas; and *Clinical Associate Professor,* Department of Medicine, University of Hawaii School of Medicine, Honolulu, Hawaii

William P. Coleman III, MD, *Clinical Associate Professor,* Department of Dermatology, Tulane University School of Medicine, New Orleans; and *Attending Dermatologist,* Doctors' Hospital of Jefferson, Metaire, Louisiana

Ralph W. Hale, MD, *Professor and Chairman,* Department of Obstetrics and Gynecology, University of Hawaii at Manoa, John A. Burns School of Medicine, Honolulu, Hawaii

Lee Hixson, MD, *Assistant Professor,* Division of Gastroenterology, Department of Medicine, University of Arizona College of Medicine, Tucson, Arizona

Victor LaCerva, MD, FAAP, *Clinical Assistant Professor,* Department of Pediatrics, University of New Mexico Medical Center; and *District Health Officer,* District II, Santa Fe, New Mexico

John Lederer, MD, *Clinical Instructor,* Department of General Internal Medicine, University of Utah Medical Center, Salt Lake City, Utah

Alvin E. Parrish, MD, FACP, *Professor,* Division of Renal Diseases, Department of Medicine, George Washington University Medical Center, Washington, DC

William Pryse-Phillips, MD, FRCP, FRCP(C), *Professor,* Division of Neurology, Department of Medicine, Memorial University of Newfoundland, Health Sciences Center, St. John's, Newfoundland, Canada

M. D. Ram,* BSc, MD, MS(Surg), PhD, FACS, FRCS(Eng), FRCS(Edin), FRCS(Can), FICS, *Professor,* Department of Surgery, Albert B. Chandler Medical Center, University of Kentucky; and *Chief,* Surgical Service, Veterans Administration Medical Center, Lexington, Kentucky

William A. Sodeman, Jr, MD, *Associate Dean for Academic Affairs,* Louisiana State University Medical Center, School of Medicine, Shreveport, Louisiana

Barry M. Stults, MD, *Associate Professor,* Department of General Internal Medicine, University of Utah Medical Center, Salt Lake City, Utah

*Deceased.

NATIONAL BOARDS EXAMINATION REVIEW

FOR PART III

1

Therapy and Management

John Lederer, MD, Lee Hixson, MD, and
Barry M. Stults, MD

DIRECTIONS: Each of the questions or incomplete statements below is followed by suggested answers or completions. Select the one that is best in each case.

1. All of the drugs listed below inhibit the metabolism of warfarin, thereby further prolonging the prothrombin time and enhancing the degree of anticoagulation except

A. cimetidine
B. trimethoprim-sulfamethoxazole
C. amiodarone
D. cholestyramine
E. sulfinpyrazone

2. Which of the following laboratory values or findings favors prerenal azotemia as the etiology of oliguria as opposed to acute tubular necrosis?

A. Urine osmolality of 250 mOsm/kg
B. Urine sodium of 50 mEq/L
C. Fractional excretion of filtered sodium < 1
D. Brown granular casts by urinalysis
E. Hematuria

3. All of the factors listed below may further decrease renal function in patients with chronic renal failure except

A. volume depletion
B. nonsteroidal antiinflammatory drugs (prostaglandin synthesis inhibitors) and aminoglycosides
C. low protein diets that meet daily minimum requirements
D. poorly controlled hypertension
E. exposure to radiocontrast materials used in diagnostic radiography

4. A 34-year-old man has the following test results on a serum total cholesterol-specimen obtained after a 12-hour fast: total cholesterol = 300 mg/dL; high density lipoprotein (HDL) cholesterol = 40 mg/dL; triglycerides = 150 mg/dL. His low density lipoprotein (LDL) cholesterol can therefore be calculated as

A. 110 mg/dL
B. 260 mg/dL
C. 150 mg/dL
D. 230 mg/dL
E. 190 mg/dL

5. A 24-year-old white man presented with a 4-week history of a 3 cm right cervical lymph node. He denied a history of fever, sweats, or weight loss, but had noted a generalized itching for 2 weeks. The remainder of the physical exam was normal. Lymph node biopsy revealed nodular sclerosing Hodgkin's disease. Subsequent work-up includes normal chest and abdomen CT scans, normal lymphangiogram, and a normal staging laparotomy. In the Ann Arbor classification for Hodgkin's disease, his disease would be

A. stage I_A
B. stage I_B
C. stage II_A
D. stage II_B
E. none of the above

6. For the patient in question 5, the expected 10-year relapse-free survival after sub–total-nodal irradiation is

A. 90%
B. 80%
C. 70%
D. 60%
E. 50%

7. The Duke's classification of colorectal cancer stratifies tumors by all of the following except

A. the degree of penetration through the bowel wall
B. the presence of lymph node metastases
C. the presence of spread to other organs
D. the degree of differentiation of the tumor

8. The most common etiology of focal or generalized seizures above the age of 50 is

A. brain tumor
B. cerebrovascular disease
C. alcoholism
D. trauma
E. brain abscess

9. True statements concerning the diagnostic evaluation of elderly patients with possible dementia include all of the following except

A. a clinical diagnosis of Alzheimer's disease can be made with 90% accuracy
B. severe depression may be mistaken for dementia
C. evaluation should usually include a CBC, metabolic screen (SMA 12-20), serum T_4, B12, VDRL, and CT or MRI brain scan
D. a toxicologic drug screen may be useful in some patients
E. multiinfarct dementia is frequently difficult to distinguish from Alzheimer's disease

10. Factors that predispose to the development of acute cholecystitis include all of the following except

- **A.** hepatitis
- **B.** cholelithiasis
- **C.** recent surgery for an unrelated disease
- **D.** burns
- **E.** trauma

11. A 45-year-old man with a 20-year history of severe chronic ethanol abuse presents to the emergency room with chief complaints of shortness of breath and epigastric abdominal pain of 24-hour duration. Physical exam is abnormal only for a BP of 90/60, a respiratory rate of 22 breaths/min that appear unusually deep, and minimal epigastric tenderness to palpation. Pertinent laboratory studies revealed: $PaO_2 = 86$; $PaCO_2 = 30$; $pH = 7.32$; $Na^+ = 140$; $K^+ = 4.5$; $Cl^- = 105$; $HCO_3 = 15$. The arterial blood gas and serum electrolyte results are consistent with which of the following acid-base disorders?

- **A.** Acute respiratory alkalosis
- **B.** Metabolic acidosis, normal anion gap variety
- **C.** Chronic respiratory alkalosis with metabolic compensation
- **D.** Metabolic acidosis, increased anion gap variety
- **E.** None of the above

12. The acid-base disorder in this patient may commonly result from

- **A.** diarrhea, renal tubular acidosis, a previous ureterosigmoidostomy surgical procedure, or primary hyperparathyroidism
- **B.** anxiety, excessive mechanical ventilation, acute asthma, or rapid ascent in altitude
- **C.** hepatic cirrhosis, pregnancy, or chronic cerebral disease (brain tumor, stroke, encephalitis, etc.)
- **D.** uncontrolled diabetes mellitus, acute and chronic alcoholism, severe acute circulatory failure, poisoning and drug toxicity, or renal failure
- **E.** none of the above

13. Helpful diagnostic studies to evaluate the acid-base disorder in this patient would include

A. urine pH, stool electrolytes, serum calcium

B. serum levels of glucose, urea nitrogen, ketones, and lactate, as well as a serum drug screen

C. serum ammonia and a computerized axial tomography (CAT) scan of the head

D. serum aldosterone

E. none of the above

14. In a woman with newly diagnosed breast cancer and palpable axillary lymph nodes, histologic evaluation fails to reveal malignancy in approximately

A. 5% of cases

B. 15% of cases

C. 25% of cases

D. 35% of cases

E. none of the above

15. The 10-year local control rate for a breast carcinoma less than 5 cm in diameter treated by excisional biopsy and primary radiotherapy is approximately

A. 90–95%

B. 80–85%

C. 70–75%

D. 60–65%

E. < 50%

16. The rhythm abnormality that is most frequently responsible for sudden cardiac death is

A. ventricular fibrillation

B. asystole

C. complete heart block

D. ventricular tachycardia

E. atrial fibrillation

17. The two most common causes of death in patients with systemic lupus erythematosus (SLE) are

- **A.** myocardial infarction and hepatic failure due to vasculitis
- **B.** cerebral infarction and status epilepticus due to vasculitis
- **C.** renal failure and superimposed infection
- **D.** respiratory failure due to acute lupus pneumonitis and pericardial tamponade
- **E.** mesenteric infarction and pancreatitis due to vasculitis

18. The two most common etiologic agents of acute bacterial arthritis in adults in the United States are

- **A.** *Neisseria gonorrhoeae* and Gram-negative aerobic bacilli
- **B.** *N. gonorrhoeae* and *Staphylococcus aureus*
- **C.** *S. aureus* and Gram-negative aerobic bacilli
- **D.** *N. gonorrhoeae* and streptococci (*Streptococcus pyogenes* and *Streptococcus pneumoniae*)
- **E.** *N. gonorrhoeae* and *Hemophilus influenzae*

19. In patients with low back pain, careful neurologic examination of the lower extremities is necessary to detect objective signs of lumbar or sacral nerve root irritation that may result from disk herniation. All of the associations below are true except

- **A.** L_4 root irritation and a decreased or absent knee jerk
- **B.** L_5 root irritation frequently causes no change in lower extremity reflexes
- **C.** S_1 root irritation and a decreased or absent ankle jerk
- **D.** S_2 to S_4 root irritation and a decreased or absent ankle jerk or an absent plantar toe response
- **E.** A positive straight leg raise is most accurate in the detection of L_3 and L_4 root irritation

20. All of the following statements about rheumatoid factor (RF) are true except

A. only 70% of patients with rheumatoid arthritis have a positive RF

B. high titers of RF in patients with rheumatoid arthritis increase the risk of severe disease and extraarticular features

C. 10% to 20% of unselected persons over age 65 have a positive RF

D. positive RF may be seen in a variety of rheumatic diseases, acute viral infections, and certain chronic lung and liver diseases

✓**E.** high levels of RF contribute directly to tissue injury in rheumatoid arthritis

21. All of the following factors increase the risk of symptomatic osteoporosis in women except

A. low initial bone density

B. premature menopause

✓**C.** a diet containing 1000–1500 mg/day of elemental calcium

D. smoking and heavy alcohol use

E. long-term intake of phenytoin or glucocorticoids

22. Which of the following diagnostic tests effectively rule out the diagnosis of active pulmonary tuberculosis?

A. Pulmonary infiltrate(s) localized to the lower lobe(s) by chest x-ray

B. Negative intermediate-strength (5 TU PPD) tuberculin test

C. Absence of acid-fast bacilli in six stained sputum specimens

D. Normal white blood cell count with normal differential

✓ **E.** None of the above

DIRECTIONS: Each group of questions below consists of lettered headings followed by a list of numbered words or statements. For each numbered word or statement, select the one lettered heading that is most closely associated with it. Each lettered heading may be selected once, more than once, or not at all.

Questions 23–26: Match the lettered compounds with the appropriate numbered consequence of inhalational exposure.

A. Asbestos
B. Silica
C. Coal dust
D. Beryllium
E. Isocyanates

23. Increased susceptibility to mycobacterial infection and disease

24. Pulmonary disease roentgenographically and histologically similar to sarcoidosis

25. Increased incidence of mesothelioma

26. Increased incidence of bronchogenic carcinoma

Questions 27–30: Match the lettered etiology of pleural effusion with the most appropriate numbered pleural fluid, serum chemistries, cell count, and differentials.

A. Congestive heart failure
B. Empyema
C. Systemic lupus erythematosus
D. Pancreatitis with pseudocyst
E. Benign asbestos-induced pleural effusion

27. Serum glucose = 100 mg/dL; pleural glucose = 98 mg/dL; serum total protein = 6.0 g/dL; pleural protein = 4.0 g/dL; serum LDH = 300 IU/L; pleural LDH = 250 IU/L; serum pH = 7.43; pleural pH = 7.44; serum amylase = 100 U/dL (normal range = 60–180 U/dL); pleural amylase = 40 U/dL; pleural C_3 complement = 30 mg/dL (normal range = 55–120 mg/dL)

28. Serum glucose = 100 mg/dL; pleural glucose = 98 mg/dL; serum total protein = 6.0 g/dL; pleural protein = 2.0 g/dL; serum LDH = 300 IU/L; pleural LDH = 100 IU/L; serum pH = 7.43; pleural pH = 7.44; serum amylase = 100 U/dL (normal range = 60–180 U/dL); pleural amylase = 40 U/dL; pleural C_3 complement = 100 mg/dL (normal range = 55–120 mg/dL)

29. Serum glucose = 100 mg/dL; pleural glucose = 98 mg/dL; serum total protein = 6.0 g/dL; pleural protein = 4.0 g/dL; serum LDH = 300 IU/L; pleural LDH = 250 IU/L; serum pH = 7.43; pleural pH = 7.44; serum amylase = 100 U/dL (normal range = 60–180 U/dL); pleural amylase = 300 U/dL; pleural C_3 complement = 100 mg/dL (normal range = 55–120 gm/dL)

30. Serum glucose = 100 mg/dL; pleural glucose = 20 mg/dL; serum total protein = 6.0 g/dL; pleural protein = 4.0 g/dL; serum LDH = 300 IU/L; pleural LDH = 250 IU/L; serum pH = 7.43; pleural pH = 6.96; serum amylase = 100 U/dL (normal range = 60–180 U/dL); pleural amylase = 40 U/dL; pleural C_3 complement = 100 mg/dL (normal range = 55–120 mg/dL)

Questions 31–34: Match the lettered gestational periods with the appropriate numbered techniques capable of establishing the presumptive diagnosis of pregnancy.

A. 20 weeks
B. 12 weeks
C. 10 weeks
D. 1 week
E. 17 weeks
F. 28 weeks

31. Auscultation of the fetus utilizing a fetoscope

32. Detection of fetal cardiac action by Doppler ultrasound

33. Palpation of the uterus above the symphysis pubis

34. Detection of the fetus by serum human chorionic gonadotropin (HCG)

Questions 35–39: Match the lettered chemotherapeutic agents with the appropriate numbered toxicity.

- **A.** Cyclophosphamide
- **B.** Bleomycin
- **C.** Vincristine
- **D.** Doxorubicin
- **E.** Cisplatin
- **F.** L-asparaginase

35. Peripheral neuropathy

36. Nephrotoxicity

37. Cardiomyopathy

38. Hemorrhagic cystitis

39. Pulmonary fibrosis

DIRECTIONS: For each of the questions or incomplete statements below, one or more of the answers or completions given is correct. Select

- **A** if only *1, 2,* and *3* are correct
- **B** if only *1* and *3* are correct
- **C** if only *2* and *4* are correct
- **D** if only *4* is correct
- **E** if all are correct

---

40. Hypocholesterolemic drugs that have been shown in controlled trials to lower the incidence of coronary heart disease in men with elevated levels of total and LDL cholesterol include

1. nicotinic acid (niacin)
2. gemfibrozil
3. bile acid sequestrants (cholestyramine)
4. lovastatin

41. Important adverse side effects of nonsteroidal antiinflammatory drugs (e.g, ibuprofen, indomethacin, etc.) include

1. reduction of diuretic efficacy in patients with hypertension and/or congestive heart failure
2. reversible acute renal failure
3. gastritis
4. nephrotic syndrome

42. Initial therapy for acute nongonococcal bacterial arthritis involving the knee should include

1. systemic antibiotics
2. systemic antibiotics *and* intraarticular antibiotics if inflammation is severe
3. frequent needle aspiration drainage of the joint
4. open surgical drainage of the knee to prevent joint destruction

43. In addition to a careful history and physical examination, the initial laboratory evaluation of patients with newly diagnosed stable hypertension should *routinely* include

1. intravenous pyelogram
2. urinalysis, serum potassium, BUN or creatinine, hematocrit, ECG
3. plasma catecholamines and aldosterone
4. serum glucose and cholesterol

44. Manifestations of diabetic autonomic neuropathy may include

1. delayed gastric emptying
2. orthostatic hypotension
3. bladder dysfunction
4. sudden death

Directions Summarized

A	B	C	D	E
1,2,3 only	1,3 only	2,4 only	4 only	all are correct

45. True statements about coronary artery bypass surgery (CABG) include
1. improved survival with CABG is limited to specific subsets of patients
2. CABG is more effective than medical therapy for relieving symptoms of angina
3. patency of grafted vessels may be protected by control of hypercholesterolemia and long-term therapy with antiplatelet agents
4. most patients undergoing CABG do not have return of angina over the subsequent decade

46. Which of the following drugs may retard the radiographic progression of rheumatoid arthritis?
1. Aspirin in doses producing a serum salicylate level of 25–30 mg/dL
2. Intramuscular (IM) gold salts
3. Corticosteroids
4. Penicillamine

47. Type I diabetes mellitus is associated with which of the following?
1. Low or immeasurable plasma insulin
2. Relative deficiency of plasma insulin
3. Tendency to develop diabetic ketoacidosis
4. Obese body habitus

48. Treatment of symptomatic *Pneumocystis carinii* infections in the immunocompromised host includes
1. supplemental oxygenation, as indicated
2. a 7-day course of trimethoprim-sulfamethoxazole
3. 10 to 21 days of pentamidine, IM or IV
4. rifampin and isoniazid

49. Potential sequelae of mitral valve prolapse include
  1. sudden death
  2. significant mitral regurgitation with ventricular dilatation
  3. endocarditis
  4. cerebral embolism

50. Felty's syndrome may be associated with which of the following abnormalities?
  1. Splenomegaly
  2. Neutropenia
  3. Recurrent infections
  4. Leg ulcers

51. Initial treatment of diabetic ketoacidosis invariably should include
  1. intravenous (IV) infusion of isotonic fluids
  2. IV sodium bicarbonate to raise the pH to near 7.40
  3. subcutaneous, IM, or IV infusion of insulin
  4. IV potassium

52. Paradoxical splitting of the second heart sound may occur with
  1. left bundle branch block
  2. atrial septal defect
  3. aortic stenosis
  4. pulmonary hypertension

53. Initial outpatient therapy for newly diagnosed SLE limited to fever and joint manifestations (arthralgia and arthritis) of mild to moderate severity might include
  1. aspirin
  2. antimalarial drugs
  3. nonsteroidal antiinflammatory drugs
  4. prednisone

54. Pheochromocytomas
  1. typically arise unilaterally in the adrenal gland
  2. are malignant in approximately 30% of cases
  3. may be bilateral
  4. present with sustained hypertension in $>$ 75% of cases

Directions Summarized

A	B	C	D	E
1,2,3 only	1,3 only	2,4 only	4 only	all are correct

55. Electrocardiographic manifestations of the sick sinus syndrome (SSS) may include

1. sinus arrest
2. paroxysmal atrial fibrillation
3. atrioventricular (AV) block
4. persistent atrial fibrillation with a slow ventricular response

56. Common etiologies of diabetes insipidus include

1. head trauma
2. sarcoidosis
3. malignancies
4. ruptured intracranial aneurysms

57. Short- or long-term mortality in selected patients with acute myocardial infarction (AMI) may be reduced by therapy with

1. thrombolytic agents
2. beta-blockers
3. aspirin
4. emergency percutaneous transluminal coronary angioplasty (PTCA)

58. Tests useful in diagnosing diabetes insipidus include

1. two or more fasting blood sugars
2. comparison of urinary osmolality after dehydration with that after the administration of vasopressin
3. a glucose tolerance test
4. hypertonic saline infusions

59. A paradoxical pulse may be seen with

1. cardiac tamponade
2. severe bronchial asthma
3. constrictive pericarditis
4. aortic regurgitation

60. The differential diagnosis of diffuse, radiologic decrease in bone mass includes

1. osteoporosis
2. multiple myeloma
3. primary hyperparathyroidism
4. osteomalacia

61. Factors associated with an increased risk of sudden cardiovascular collapse and death include

1. severe coronary artery disease
2. left ventricular dysfunction
3. repetitive ventricular ectopic beats (couplets and ventricular tachycardia)
4. cigarette smoking, hypercholesterolemia, hypertension, ECG evidence of left ventricular hypertrophy, diabetes mellitus, and obesity

62. Complications associated with the use of oral contraceptives include

1. thromboembolic stroke
2. pulmonary embolus
3. hypertension
4. breast cancer

63. Organisms commonly implicated in neonatal sepsis include

1. *E. coli*
2. *Neisseria meningitidis*
3. group B streptococci
4. *H. influenzae*

64. Which of the following statements concerning patients with syncope is (are) true?

1. Twenty-four-hour ambulatory ECG monitoring and intracardiac electrophysiologic studies are the most useful diagnostic tests
2. The etiology of syncope can be determined in less than 50% of patients
3. Cardiac arrhythmias are the most common cause of syncope in the general population
4. The 1-year incidence of sudden death in patients with a cardiac cause of syncope is up to 25%

Directions Summarized

A	B	C	D	E
1,2,3 only	1,3 only	2,4 only	4 only	all are correct

65. Hyponatremia due to the syndrome of inappropriate antidiuretic hormone secretion (SIADH) may be caused by which of the following drugs?

1. Oral hypoglycemic drugs tolbutamide and chlorpropamide
2. Clofibrate
3. Chemotherapeutic drugs vincristine and cyclophosphamide
4. Lithium carbonate

66. Potential side effects of thiazide diuretics include

1. hyperuricemia
2. hyperglycemia
3. hypokalemia
4. hyponatremia

67. Ascites may be associated with which of the following?

1. Myxedema
2. Constrictive pericarditis
3. Meigs' syndrome
4. Budd-Chiari syndrome

68. Typical angina pectoris in the absence of coronary artery disease may be secondary to which of the following?

1. Hypertrophic cardiomyopathy
2. Aortic stenosis
3. Pulmonary hypertension
4. Atrial myxoma

69. Asymptomatic bacteriuria occurring during pregnancy

1. occurs in up to 12% of pregnant women
2. rarely progresses to symptomatic infection
3. results in symptomatic urinary tract infection in approximately 25% of patients
4. should not be treated due to the potential adverse effects of antibiotics on the fetus

70. Which of the following statements concerning eclampsia is (are) true?
   1. The diagnosis is established by the presence of seizures alone in a pregnant woman
   2. It is thought to be secondary to intense vasospasm
   3. It rarely occurs during the first pregnancy
   4. It occurs after 20-weeks gestation

71. Which of the following statements regarding contraction stress testing is (are) true?
   1. A positive test is characterized by consistent, persistent deceleration of the fetal heart rate after the onset of uterine contractions
   2. Contraction stress testing may be contraindicated in threatened preterm delivery
   3. An adequate test may require IV oxytocin
   4. A positive test represents aortocaval compression by the pregnant uterus

72. Human retroviruses
   1. have been identified since the early 1900s
   2. are RNA viruses
   3. have a genome comprised of DNA
   4. have been implicated in the acquired immunodeficiency syndrome (AIDS)

73. Patients at relatively high risk for infective endocarditis include
   1. patients with transvenous cardiac pacemakers
   2. patients with prosthetic heart valves
   3. patients with atrial septal defects
   4. patients with mitral insufficiency

74. Carcinoembryonic antigen (CEA) may be elevated in
   1. colorectal cancer
   2. alcoholic cirrhosis
   3. breast cancer
   4. testicular cancer

Directions Summarized

A	B	C	D	E
1,2,3 only	1,3 only	2,4 only	4 only	all are correct

75. Sickle cell anemia

1. is found in approximately 8% of black Americans
2. is associated with aseptic necrosis of the femoral head
3. should maintain a hematocrit of approximately 35 by the judicious use of transfusions
4. may present in sickle crisis as a seizure, stroke, or in coma

76. A 50-year-old white man presents with a several-year history of progressive increase in shoe size and enlargement of the tongue. Abnormalities that might be encountered in the evaluation of this patient would commonly include

1. elevated growth hormone level
2. glucose intolerance
3. enlarged sella turcica
4. lack of growth hormone response to thyrotropin-releasing hormone (TRH)

77. Factors thought to be of etiologic importance in the development of hepatocellular carcinoma include

1. hemochromatosis
2. aflatoxins
3. chronic hepatitis B infection
4. long-term estrogen therapy

78. Indications for annual mammography include

1. history of prior breast cancer
2. patients with a sibling with breast cancer
3. patients whose mother had breast cancer
4. patients over 40 years of age

79. A 45-year-old white man presents with a 6-month history of fatigue. Physical exam is remarkable for a BP of 160/100 and multiple abdominal striae. Administration of 1 mg of dexamethasone at midnight results in an 8:00 AM plasma cortisol of 10 mg/100 mL (normal $<$ 5 mg/100 mL). The differential diagnosis includes

1. Cushing's disease
2. chronic alcoholism
3. obesity
4. chronic endogenous depression

80. Subsequent testing in this patient reveals the failure of the plasma cortisol to suppress to $<$ 50% of control values after 2 mg of dexamethasone every 6 hours for 48 hours. The most likely etiology(ies) of this patient's disorder would be

1. pituitary microadenoma
2. ectopic adrenocorticotropic hormone (ACTH) production
3. morbid obesity
4. adrenal neoplasm

81. The patient is found to have a normal value for urine 17-ketosteroids and a normal CT scan of the abdomen. In this patient

1. plasma ACTH levels are often elevated
2. adrenal carcinoma is very likely
3. the most likely diagnosis is a small cell carcinoma of the lungs
4. abdominal exploration is indicated

82. A 56-year-old white man with a prior splenectomy is admitted to the intensive care unit for pneumococcal sepsis. Physical exam is unremarkable except for a questionable delayed relaxation of the deep tendon reflexes. Serum T3 is decreased. The differential diagnosis would include

1. hypothyroidism
2. increased concentration of thyroxin-binding globulins
3. the "low-T3 syndrome" (euthyroid sick syndrome)
4. Graves' disease

Directions Summarized

A	B	C	D	E
1,2,3 only	1,3 only	2,4 only	4 only	all are correct

83. A 30-year-old white male homosexual presents with a 6-week history of watery diarrhea, abdominal cramping, and weight loss. Etiologies would include
1. *Shigella*
2. cryptosporidiosis
3. *Salmonella*
4. *Isospora belli*

84. Initial evaluation of the patient in Question 83 would include
1. stool culture and sensitivity
2. Ziehl-Neelsen preparation of the stool
3. wet preparation of the stool
4. intestinal biopsy

85. Physiologic consequences of normal aging include
1. significant reduction in glomerular filtration rate (GFR)
2. reduction in hemoglobin concentration to 11–13 g/dL for men and to 10–12 g/dL for women
3. significant reduction in the ventilatory function of the lung
4. elevation of the fasting blood glucose to 140–160 mg%

86. Common causes of upper gastrointestinal bleeding include
1. peptic ulceration
2. Mallory-Weiss syndrome
3. variceal bleeding
4. gastric carcinoma

87. True statements concerning the symptoms of transient ischemic attacks (TIA) include
   1. amaurosis fugax suggests carotid TIA
   2. syncope not associated with focal neurologic symptoms is usually due to vertebrobasilar TIA
   3. transient bilateral visual blurring and bilateral motor or sensory symptoms suggest vertebrobasilar TIA
   4. recurrent episodic vertigo not associated with focal neurologic symptoms is usually due to vertebrobasilar TIA

88. Criteria for the diagnosis of brain death include
   1. absence of cerebral and brain stem function
   2. known etiology and duration of coma with depressant drug poisoning explicitly ruled out
   3. EEG isoelectric ("flat") for 30 minutes at maximal gain
   4. absence of all spinal reflexes

89. Known etiologies of parkinsonism include
   1. multiple small cerebral infarctions
   2. reserpine
   3. phenothiazines and butyrophenones
   4. bromocriptine

90. A 30-year-old woman presents with a BP of 190/110 and a serum potassium of 2.8. Possible etiologies for her hypertension would include
   1. primary aldosteronism
   2. salt-wasting nephropathy
   3. Cushing's syndrome
   4. renovascular hypertension

91. A patient complaining of long-standing heartburn undergoes esophagoscopy, and a mucosal biopsy of the distal esophagus reveals columnar mucosa. The patient is at increased risk for developing
   1. adenocarcinoma of the esophagus
   2. esophageal ulcers
   3. peptic stricture
   4. achalasia

Directions Summarized

A	B	C	D	E
1,2,3 only	1,3 only	2,4 only	4 only	all are correct

92. A 38-year-old man presents with a gnawing epigastric pain that he has noted to be relieved by eating and antacids. Upper endoscopy is performed and reveals a 1.5 cm ulcer in the duodenal bulb. Appropriate initial therapy might include

1. antacids
2. H_2 receptor antagonists
3. sucralfate
4. partial gastrectomy

93. Diarrhea that is associated with arthritis may be seen in

1. Crohn's disease
2. Whipple's disease
3. Yersinia enterocolitica enteritis
4. Zollinger-Ellison syndrome

94. Delay in gastric emptying without obstruction may be seen with

1. diabetes mellitus
2. gastric malignancy
3. anticholinergic drugs
4. metoclopramide

95. Abundant white blood cells in a stool specimen may be seen with

1. ulcerative colitis
2. giardiasis
3. radiation enteritis
4. irritable bowel syndrome

96. Which of the associations listed below are true concerning potential side effects of psychoactive drugs?

1. tricyclic antidepressants: orthostatic hypotension, advanced heart block, ventricular arrhythmias
2. lithium: orthostatic hypotension, obstructive jaundice, tardive dyskinesia
3. benzodiazepines: withdrawal seizures, paradoxical aggressive behavior, excessive sedation when combined with other CNS depressants
4. neuroleptic (antipsychotic) medications: hypothyroidism, nephrogenic diabetes insipidus, toxic serum levels with concurrent diuretic therapy

97. A patient with acute renal failure is found to have a serum potassium of 6.8 mEq/L. Further diagnostic studies needed emergently include which of the following?

1. serum blood urea nitrogen (BUN) and creatinine
2. serum magnesium
3. serum calcium
4. ECG

98. Therapy that may ameliorate life-threatening cardiotoxicity from hyperkalemia within 30 to 60 minutes or less include(s)

1. IV administration of 10 U of regular insulin and 25 g of glucose
2. IV administration of 10 mL of 10% calcium gluconate over 5 to 10 minutes
3. IV administration of 50–100 mEq of sodium bicarbonate
4. oral administration of 50–100 g Kayexalate in 20 mL of 70% sorbitol

99. Which systolic murmur(s) may increase in intensity and/or duration with a postural change from the lying to standing positions?

1. hypertrophic obstructive cardiomyopathy
2. aortic stenosis
3. mitral valve prolapse
4. mitral regurgitation

Directions Summarized

A	B	C	D	E
1,2,3 only	1,3 only	2,4 only	4 only	All are correct

100. A 30-year-old IV drug abuser presents with a 2-day history of headaches, fever, and altered mental status. Evaluation might include

1. brain biopsy
A **2.** CT or MRI scan of the brain
3. lumbar puncture
4. cerebral angiogram

Explanatory Answers

1. D. Coadministration of cholestyramine (a hypolipidemic agent) with warfarin can decrease the absorption of warfarin and result in a subtherapeutic prothrombin time in patients with previously adequate anticoagulation. The addition of concurrent therapy with cimetidine, trimethoprim-sulfamethoxazole, amiodarone, sulfinpyrazone, and a number of other drugs to patients taking warfarin inhibits warfarin metabolism and may result in serious overanticoagulation and hemorrhage. A large number of drugs interact with warfarin, and significant caution is required when adding or subtracting any drug from the regimen of a patient taking warfarin. (Ref. 2, pp. 99–101)

2. C. Prerenal azotemia is typically associated with a urine osmolality > 500 mOsm/kg, urine sodium < 20 mEq/L, and a fractional excretion of sodium (FeNa) < 1.

$$\text{FeNa} = \frac{\text{Urine Na/serum Na}}{\text{Urine creatinine/serum creatinine}}$$

a urine osmolality < 400 mOsm/kg, urine sodium > 40 mEq/L, brown granular casts on urinalysis, and an FeNa > 2 are consistent with a diagnosis of acute tubular necrosis. Hematuria may be associated with a variety of renal and urologic disorders. (Ref. 1, p. 1152)

3. C. A low protein diet that meets minimum daily requirements (0.6 grams protein per kilogram of body weight per day) will decrease azotemia, improve symptoms, and possibly slow the rate of decline in renal function in patients with chronic renal failure. Volume depletion, toxic drug therapy, exposure to radiocontrast dye, and uncontrolled hypertension must be avoided or detected early and corrected in these patients to prevent progressive loss of renal function. (Ref. 2, pp. 569–572)

4. D. The total cholesterol equals the sum of the LDL cholesterol, HDL cholesterol, and VLDL cholesterol. When serum triglycerides are ≤ 400 mg/dL, the VLDL cholesterol can be estimated as the triglyceride value divided by 5. Therefore, LDL cholesterol = total cholesterol − (HDL cholesterol + triglyceride/5), or LDL cholesterol = 300 mg/dL − (40 + 150/5) = 230 mg/dL. The level of LDL cholesterol is causally related to the risk of coronary heart disease, and lowering elevated LDL cholesterol levels reduces the incidence of coronary heart disease. Therapeutic decisions should be made according to the level of LDL cholesterol rather than the total cholesterol. (Ref. 22, pp. 37, 40, 44)

5. A. Involvement of a single lymph node region is classified as stage I. Stage II disease is involvement of two or more lymph node regions on the same side of the diaphragm. Involvement of lymph node regions on both sides of the diaphragm (stage III) or diffuse involvement of an extralymphatic organ (stage IV) is associated with a poorer prognosis. Fever > 38°C, sweats, or weight loss > 10% are designated as "B" symptoms. (Ref. 8, p. 1648)

6. A. Results of treatment for stage I_A Hodgkin's disease at the Joint Center for Radiation Therapy have yielded a survival of 95%, with a relapse-free survival of 91%. For patients with stage II_A disease, treatment with sub–total-nodal irradiation results in relapse-free survival, and survival, of 79 and 93%, respectively. For stage III_A disease, the corresponding figures are 68% and 40%. Stages III_B and IV are generally treated with systemic chemotherapy. (Ref. 8, pp. 1663–1665)

7. D. According to the Duke's classification, stage A tumors are limited to the mucosa and submucosa, while a stage B tumor is confined to the bowel wall. Spread to regional lymph nodes (stage C) or to other organs (stage D) results in a lower 5-year survival. Although less differentiated tumors tend to be more invasive, histologic criteria are not part of the classification. (Ref. 1, p. 1300)

8. B. New onset generalized or focal seizures in persons over 50 years of age most commonly result from cerebrovascular disease, especially as a late sequel to cerebral thrombosis, embolus, or hemorrhage; less frequently, these disorders may present acutely with a seizure. Brain tumors are the second most common cause of seizures in this age group. In young adults ages 18 to 35, prior head trauma, alcoholism, and brain tumors are the most common causes of seizures. (Ref. 1, pp. 1924, 1925)

9. E. Multiinfarct dementia from cerebrovascular disease, the cause of 20% of progressive dementias, is usually easily differentiated from Alzheimer's disease by its stuttering progression, focal motor symptoms and signs, and the presence of multiple infarctions on a CT or MRI brain scan. Alzheimer's disease, the cause of 50% to 60% of dementias, can be diagnosed with 90% accuracy using history, physical examination, and the laboratory tests listed in C; a careful drug history, occasionally supplemented by a toxicologic drug screen, will rule out chronic drug intoxication. A careful history and examination are needed to rule out depression, which may mimic dementia or complicate and exacerbate it. (Ref. 2, pp. 2088, 2089; Ref. 6, 13:VII:1)

10. A. About 95% of patients with acute cholecystitis have gallstones (cholelithiasis), while 5% do not. Risk factors for acalculous cholecystitis include recent major surgery, trauma, or burns, and perhaps childbirth and a variety of debilitating diseases. Nearly 50% of cases have no precipitating factor. Hepatitis is not known to be a risk factor. (Ref. 18, pp. 1138–1145)

11. D. The patient demonstrates acidemia, hypocapnia, and an elevated anion gap [anion gap $= Na^+ - (Cl^- + HCO_3^-)$] of 20 mEq/L (normally 10–12 mEq/L). These values are consistent with a metabolic acidosis, increased anion gap variety. Acute respiratory alkalosis would be associated with a normal anion gap, an elevated arterial pH = 7.48–7.50, and an $HCO_3^- = 23$. Chronic respiratory alkalosis with metabolic compensation would demonstrate a normal anion gap, an elevated arterial pH = 7.42, and an $HCO_3^- = 21$. (Ref. 2, pp. 551–558)

12. D. Metabolic acidosis with an increased anion gap may result from diabetic ketoacidosis, alcoholic ketoacidosis, lactic acidosis from circulatory failure, certain poisons and drug toxicity (salicylates, ethylene glycol, methanol) or renal failure. The disorders listed in **A**, **B**, and **C** may produce normal anion gap metabolic acidosis, acute respiratory alkalosis, and chronic respiratory alkalosis, respectively. (Ref. 1, pp. 210–214)

13. B. Serum glucose, urea nitrogen, ketones, lactate, and a serum drug screen for salicylates, ethylene glycol, and methanol are all useful tests to assess the etiology of increased anion gap metabolic acidosis. The studies listed in **A**, **C**, and **D** might help assess the etiology of an undiagnosed normal anion gap metabolic acidosis, chronic respiratory alkalosis, and metabolic alkalosis, respectively. (Ref. 1, pp. 208–214)

14. C. Physical examination yields a false-positive (enlarged nodes that are histologically negative) rate of approximately 25% in breast cancer patients with palpable axillary nodes. Similarly, in the absence of adenopathy on physical exam, pathologic examination reveals metastatic tumor in approximately 30% of cases (false-negative). The presence of histologically involved lymph nodes is the most powerful predictor of future recurrence. (Ref. 8, pp. 1124, 1125)

15. A. Multiple retrospective and prospective studies have shown excellent control of the primary tumor in stage I ($<$ 2 cm) and stage II (2–5 cm) breast cancer. Long-term survival is equivalent to that obtained by modified radical mastectomy. (Ref. 8, pp. 1142–1146)

16. A. Ventricular fibrillation is by far the most common rhythm abnormality found in patients monitored shortly after sudden cardiovascular collapse. Ventricular tachycardia may precede ventricular fibrillation in an unknown percentage of patients. Bradyarrhythmias such as asystole and complete heart block are found less frequently. Atrial fibrillation is not responsible for sudden cardiac death. (Ref. 9, pp. 752–755)

17. C. Renal failure and superimposed infection are the most common causes of death in SLE. Central nervous system disease, including major stroke and status epilepticus, is the third ranked cause of death. Acute lupus pneumonitis, pericardial tamponade, mesenteric infarction, pancreatitis, and myocardial ischemia are less frequent complications of SLE. Hepatic failure is not a complication of SLE. (Ref. 12, pp. 53, 58)

18. B. *N. gonorrhoeae* accounts for two thirds to three fourths of all acute bacterial arthritis in adults in the United States. The causes of acute nongonococcal bacterial arthritis include *S. aureus* (65% of cases), *Streptococcus pyogenes* and *Streptococcus pneumoniae* (15%–20% of cases), and Gram-negative aerobic bacilli (15% of cases). *H. influenzae* septic arthritis in adults is less common, but may be increasing in prevalence. (Ref. 13, pp. 1515, 1516)

19. E. A positive straight leg raise test (induction of pain in a radicular distribution in the lower extremity when the leg is lifted by the heel with the knee fully extended) is most accurate in detecting lesions (eg, herniated disks) that irritate the L_5 and S_1 roots. A negative straight leg raise test effectively excludes disk herniation in patients less than age 30. (Ref. 13, p. 451)

20. E. RF does not cause the inflammation of rheumatoid arthritis; some healthy, asymptomatic persons have RF in their serum. It is important to note that RF is neither sensitive nor specific for the diagnosis of rheumatoid arthritis; up to 30% of rheumatoid arthritis patients do not have RF, while healthy individuals and persons with other rheumatic disorders or unrelated diseases may have detectable titers in their serum. The diagnosis of rheumatoid arthritis is determined primarily by clinical presentation rather than by the presence or absence of RF. (Ref. 1, p. 1425; Ref. 2, p. 1995)

21. C. It is recommended that all premenopausal and postmenopausal women consume 1000–1500 mg/day of elemental calcium; however, the average calcium intake of postmenopausal American women is only 550 mg/day. The low initial bone density of white and Asian women increases their risk of osteoporosis as compared with black women. The estrogen deficiency of premature menopause results in earlier onset of osteoporosis. Smoking, heavy alcohol intake, and chronic phenytoin and glucocorticoid therapy are other important risk factors. Prophylactic or preventive therapy with estrogen will have the greatest benefit/toxicity ratio in high-risk individuals. (Ref. 2, pp. 1511, 1514, 1515)

22. E. While reactivation pulmonary tuberculosis most commonly appears in the apical and posterior segments of the upper lobes, primary pulmonary tuberculosis infection and disease commonly develop in the lower lobes. Of patients with active pulmonary tuberculosis, 15%–20% may have false-negative intermediate-strength tuberculin tests. Sputum smears for acid-fast bacilli are frequently negative in patients who are not discharging large numbers of tuberculous organisms even though subsequent cultures are positive. The white blood cell count may be elevated, normal, or low in patients with tuberculosis. (Ref. 1, pp. 627, 629, 630)

23. B. Patients with silicosis are at increased risk to develop infec-
24. D. tions with both *Mycobacterium tuberculosis* and atypical
25. A. mycobacteria. Beryllium may produce a chronic, granulo-
26. A. matous, interstitial lung disease difficult to distinguish
from sarcoidosis. Asbestos exposure is associated with an increased incidence of both mesothelioma and bronchogenic carcinoma (squamous and adenocarcinoma cell types). Isolated exposure to coal dust is not associated with any of the listed consequences. Isocyanates used in the plastics industry may result in occupational asthma in some susceptible workers. (Ref. 1, pp. 1070, 1071; Ref. 2, p. 2358)

27. C. The diagnostic approach to pleural effusions requires con-
28. A. sideration of the patient's clinical presentation in conjunc-
29. D. tion with biochemical and often cytologic and microbio-
30. B. logic analysis of pleural fluid. The pleural fluid should first
be categorized as transudative or exudative. Transudates demonstrate (1) pleural protein: serum total protein ratio <0.5; (2) pleural LDH: serum LDH ratio <0.6; (3) absolute pleural LDH <200 IU/L. The pleural fluid is an exudate if any of the above three criteria are not met. According to these criteria, the pleural fluid in question 28 is a transudate while the pleural fluids in questions 27, 29, and 30 are exudates. The most common cause of a pleural transudate is congestive heart failure; other causes include nephrotic syndrome and cirrhosis with ascites. Exudative effusions require further cytologic, microbiologic, and biochemical evaluation. Pleural pH <7.20 and pleural glucose <60 mg% may be seen with empyema, malignancy, rheumatoid arthritis, and esophageal rupture; microbiologic studies (positive bacterial culture) and the patient's clinical presentation are required to confirm that the pleural fluid in question 30 is an empyema. Pleural amylase >200 U/dL may be seen in patients with pancreatic disease, malignancy, and esophageal rupture; further studies are needed to determine the diagnosis in the patient in question 29. Low pleural fluid complement may be seen in patients with lupus erythematosus and rheumatoid arthritis. Asbestos exposure may produce an exudative pleural effusion with normal glucose, pH, amylase, and complement. (Ref. 2, pp. 467, 468, 2362)

31. E. The serum HCG level rises 1 week prior to the expected
32. C. menses following fertilization. Doppler ultrasound and

33. B. auscultation detect evidence of the fetus at the times stated.
34. D. At 12 and 20 weeks of gestation, the uterus may be palpated at the level of the symphysis pubis and umbilicus, respectively. (Ref. 10, pp. 211, 212, 249)

35. C. Vincristine is associated with peripheral neuropathy, mar-
36. E. row suppression, and the syndrome of inappropriate anti-
37. D. diuretic hormone secretion (SIADH). The major toxic ef-
38. A. fects of cisplatin are gastrointestinal, renal, and otologic.
39. B. Renal toxicity is attenuated by concomitant administration of IV fluids and mannitol. Doxorubicin is associated with two variants of cardiac toxicity. The first is an acute transient one consisting of ST-T wave changes and arrhythmias. The second is a chronic, dose-related cardiomyopathy seen in less than 3% of patients receiving a total dose of less than 500 mg/m^2 of body surface area. Cyclophosphamide is associated with hemorrhagic cystitis, alopecia, and marrow suppression. Acutely, it is associated with nausea and vomiting. Bleomycin administration is associated with pulmonary toxicity. Toxicity generally occurs at a cumulative dose of greater than 400 U. (Ref. 8, pp. 288, 289)

40. A. Nicotinic acid, bile acid sequestrants (cholestyramine and colestipol), and gemfibrozil have all been shown to lower the incidence of coronary heart disease in controlled clinical trials of men with elevated levels of total and LDL cholesterol. There is a 2% reduction in cardiac mortality for each 1% reduction in total cholesterol. The long-term safety of nicotinic acid and bile acid sequestrants has also been demonstrated, and these are considered the drugs of choice for most patients. Lovastatin, a recently released HMG-CoA reductase inhibitor, effectively lowers LDL cholesterol, but studies on its efficacy in reducing coronary heart disease and long-term safety are not yet available. (Ref. 22, pp. 38, 55)

41. E. Nonsteroidal antiinflammatory agents are widely prescribed and are associated with significant adverse reactions in certain patient groups. They blunt the natriuretic (sodium diuresis) response to thiazide and loop diuretics and may thereby increase sodium retention and exacerbate hypertension and heart failure. They may precipitate acute renal failure, including hyperkalemia and metabolic acidosis, in patients dependent on prostaglandin synthesis for maintenance of intrarenal blood flow (patients with congestive heart failure, cirrhosis with ascites, underlying renal disease, and in the elderly). They occasionally cause acute interstitial nephritis with nephrotic syndrome and both acute and chronic gastritis. (Ref. 2, pp. 232, 234, 608, 609, 689)

42. B. Systemic antibiotics and frequent (up to several times per day) needle aspiration drainage of the joint are adequate initial therapy for most cases of acute nongonococcal bacterial arthritis. Intraarticular administration of antibiotics is not required and may induce a chemical synovitis. Open surgical drainage is required only for bacterial arthritis of the hip or for joints with chronic infection and loculated pus. (Ref. 1, p. 1463)

43. C. An adequate laboratory evaluation for the vast majority of patients with hypertension includes an ECG and creatinine or BUN to screen for cardiac and renal end-organ damage, a urinalysis, creatinine, and potassium to screen for the infrequently found (less than 5%) secondary causes of hypertension, and a serum cholesterol and glucose to screen for other cardiovascular risk factors whose copresence greatly increases the individual risk to the patient. Other expensive diagnostic tests, such as IV pyelograms, renal arteriograms, or hormonal studies, are indicated only when the history, physical examination, or routine laboratory tests suggest the possible existence of secondary causes of hypertension. Some clinicians would also further evaluate hypertensives under age 30 and patients with poorly controlled or suddenly worsened hypertension. (Ref. 2, p. 282; Ref. 6, 1:VII:5–7)

44. E. All are presentations of diabetic autonomic neuropathy. Other manifestations include dysphagia, diarrhea, impotence, and retrograde ejaculation. (Ref. 1, pp. 1792, 1793)

45. A. Improved survival with CABG as compared with medical therapy has been documented for patients with left main and/or three vessel coronary artery stenoses associated with left ventricular dysfunction; whether mortality is reduced in some other subsets of angina patients is controversial. Angina is completely relieved for months to years in two thirds of patients and improved in most of the others. Hypolipidemic therapy in patients with hypercholesterolemia retards the progression of atherosclerosis in grafted and native vessels, and antiplatelet therapy with aspirin helps prevent graft closure. CABG is palliative rather than curative therapy, and most patients eventually redevelop angina. (Ref. 2, pp. 328, 337–339)

46. C. Although each of these drugs may relieve some of the signs and symptoms of rheumatoid arthritis, only gold and penicillamine have been shown to retard radiographic joint destruction. (Ref. 12, pp. 46–48, 192)

47. B. Type I diabetes mellitus, also known as insulin-dependent diabetes mellitus, is characterized by low to immeasurable plasma insulin levels and the tendency to develop diabetic ketoacidosis. In contrast, in type II, or noninsulin-dependent diabetes mellitus, plasma insulin levels are normal to high in absolute terms. However, they are lower than expected for the plasma glucose. An obese body habitus is associated with type II diabetes mellitus. (Ref. 1, p. 1782)

48. B. Pneumocystis infection presents as dyspnea, cough, tachypnea, and chest tightness with perihilar infiltrates on chest radiograph. A minimum of 14 days of trimethoprim-sulfamethoxazole is considered the treatment of choice. For patients unresponsive to 7 to 10 days of trimethoprim-sulfamethoxazole, or who are otherwise unable to tolerate it, 10 to 21 days of pentamidine is equally effective. The role of supplemental oxygenation in pulmonary infections should always be determined. Rifampin and isoniazid are effective antituberculosis agents, but have not been found to be of benefit in pneumocystis pneumonia. (Ref. 2, pp. 1879–1881, 1686, 1687)

49. E. The majority of patients with mitral valve prolapse are asymptomatic with an excellent prognosis. A small percentage of patients may experience one or more of the listed complications. (Ref. 11, pp. 184, 185, 1358)

50. E. Felty's syndrome consists of chronic rheumatoid arthritis in association with splenomegaly and neutropenia. These patients may be troubled with recurrent infections and leg ulcers. (Ref. 12, p. 44)

51. B. After establishing the diagnosis of diabetic ketoacidosis, insulin and infusion of IV 0.9% NaCl should be administered. Sodium bicarbonate should be reserved for severely acidotic patients, and then the pH should be corrected only partially. In the majority of patients, potassium should be reserved until urine output is documented. (Ref. 1, pp. 1788, 1789)

52. B. Paradoxical splitting of the second heart sound is usually secondary to left-sided electrical or mechanical emptying delay, as occurs with left bundle branch block or aortic stenosis. Atrial septal defect typically produces a fixed splitting of the second heart sound. In pulmonary hypertension, the second heart sound usually splits normally. (Ref. 11, pp. 166–176).

53. B. Aspirin in full antiinflammatory dosage is the initial drug therapy for fever and joint manifestations of SLE; nonsteroidal antiinflammatory agents may be used if aspirin is poorly tolerated. Antimalarial drugs or prednisone should be reserved for patients who fail to respond to initial therapy. (Ref. 12, p. 57)

54. B. Pheochromocytomas are tumors that arise 90% of the time in the adrenal gland. Approximately 10% of cases may be bilateral, while $< 10\%$ are malignant. Sixty percent have sustained hypertension, with the other 40% having increased blood pressure during attacks consisting of headaches, profuse sweating, palpitations, apprehension, and pain in the chest or abdomen. (Ref. 1, p. 1775)

55. E. SSS may be associated with abnormalities of impulse formation in the sinus node, atrial tachyarrhythmias, and delayed impulse conduction through the AV node and His-Purkinje system. (Ref. 11, pp. 449, 450)

56. B. Idiopathic causes, trauma, pituitary surgery, and malignancy account for 80%–90% of cases of diabetes insipidus. Sarcoid and ruptured intracranial aneurysms are each implicated in 1% of cases. (Ref. 1, p. 1725)

57. A. Thrombolytic therapy with intracoronary or IV streptokinase or tissue plasminogen-activator reduces infarct size and mortality when given to patients with anterior Q wave AMI within 2 to 3 hours of the onset of symptoms. Long-term therapy with certain oral beta blockers (propranolol, metoprolol, and timolol) can reduce mortality and reinfarction in selected patients during at least the first 3 years after AMI. Aspirin 300 mg/day may also reduce the incidence of recurrent coronary events in some AMI survivors. Emergency PTCA has not been proven to reduce mortality from AMI. (Ref. 2, pp. 334, 335)

58. C. In contrast to normal subjects, the maximal urinary osmolality after dehydration will increase by greater than 9% with the injection of vasopressin. With hypertonic saline infusions, most patients with diabetes insipidus display no decrease in free water clearance as plasma osmolality exceeds 300 mosm/kg. Fasting blood sugars and glucose tolerance tests are useful in diagnosing diabetes mellitus, not diabetes insipidus. (Ref. 1, pp. 1726, 1727)

59. A. A paradoxical pulse denotes a greater than 10 mmHg inspiratory decrease in systolic arterial pressure, and its presence in the setting of hypotension suggests cardiac tamponade. It can occasionally occur in patients with constrictive pericarditis, restrictive cardiomyopathy, chronic obstructive pulmonary disease, shock, and asthma. Aortic regurgitation is associated with a widened pulse pressure but not with a paradoxical pulse. (Ref. 9, p. 24)

60. E. A radiologic decrease in skeletal mass (osteopenia) can be produced by all of the listed entities. Osteomalacia may present with distinct radiologic signs, but frequently demonstrates only nonspecific osteopenia. Patients with bone pain or fractures associated with osteopenia should be thoroughly evaluated for all of these disorders as well as for the different etiologies and types of osteoporosis. (Ref. 1, pp. 1890–1892)

61. E. Severe, multivessel coronary artery disease is found at autopsy in 75% of patients with sudden death. Severe left ventricular dysfunction and repetitive ventricular ectopy increase the risk of sudden death, especially when both are present; ventricular arrhythmias alone are associated with a lesser risk of sudden death when they are not accompanied by left ventricular dysfunction or acute ischemia. Presence of coronary risk factors and left ventricular hypertrophy also increase the risk of sudden death. (Ref. 1, pp. 158, 159)

62. A. There is a three- to nine-fold increased risk for thromboembolic stroke in women taking oral contraceptives. Up to a twelve-fold increased risk for deep vein thrombosis and pulmonary embolism has been reported. Approximately 5% of women taking oral contraceptives develop hypertension. There is no increased risk for breast cancer. (Ref. 1, pp. 1832–1834)

63. B. The pathogens most frequently responsible for neonatal sepsis are group B streptococci and *E. coli.*, accounting for 50% of cases in some hospitals. *H. influenzae* and *N. meningitidis* are most frequently implicated in the older infant and child. (Ref. 7, p. 480)

64. C. A careful history and physical examination are clearly the most useful diagnostic tests to evaluate patients with syncope; the yield of other tests is much lower. Twenty-four hour ambulatory ECG monitoring and intracardiac electrophysiologic evaluation with programmed atrial and ventricular stimulation may detect cardiac arrhythmias as the cause of otherwise unexplained syncope, especially if the syncope is recurrent and/or the patient has structural heart disease. Without appropriate treatment, patients with a cardiac cause of syncope (eg, arrhythmias or valvular heart disease) have a 25% incidence of sudden death after 1 year. Despite extensive evaluation, no diagnosis is made in more than 50% of patients with syncope. (Ref. 9, pp. 890, 892, 893)

65. A. Tolbutamide, chlorpropamide, clofibrate, vincristine, cyclophosphamide, haloperidol, thioridazine, carbamazepine, and amitriptyline may all precipitate hyponatremia by stimulating inappropriate secretion of ADH (antidiuretic hormone) and/or by potentiating the effects of already circulating ADH with a resultant decrease in free water clearance. Lithium carbonate may interfere with the renal action of ADH, and thereby cause nephrogenic diabetes insipidus and hypernatremia. (Ref. 1, pp. 201, 2102)

66. E. Precipitation or exacerbation of hyperuricemia, hyperglycemia, hypokalemia, and hyponatremia may each occur with thiazide diuretic therapy; thiazides may also increase serum cholesterol. (Ref. 1, pp. 201, 1031)

67. E. Profound hypothyroidism may be associated with pericardial and pleural effusions, in addition to ascites. Budd-Chiari syndrome (inferior vena cava or hepatic vein obstruction) and constrictive pericarditis may result in elevated portal pressures secondary to passive hepatic congestion. Meigs' syndrome consists of hydrothorax and ascites with benign ovarian tumors. (Ref. 1, pp. 188–190, 1348, 1349)

68. A. Angina pectoris without coronary atherosclerosis may occur in each of these three disorders. It may also occur with coronary artery spasm and aortic regurgitation. Atrial myxomas are not associated with anginal chest pain. (Ref. 2, pp. 323, 324)

69. B. The incidence of asymptomatic bacteriuria ranges from 2% to 12% and progresses to symptomatic infection in approximately 25% of patients. Asymptomatic bacteriuria should be treated during pregnancy. (Ref. 10, p. 583).

70. C. The symptoms of preeclampsia include the presence of increased blood pressure, sudden weight gain, headaches, and visual disturbances. Eclampsia is diagnosed by the presence of seizures, in addition to any of the abnormalities of preeclampsia. Vasospasm is felt to be the basis of the disease. Nulliparity is a major predisposing factor. Preeclampsia-eclampsia occurs after 20-weeks gestation. (Ref. 10, pp. 540–545)

71. A. A positive contraction stress test is indicated by consistent, persistent deceleration of the fetal heart rate after the onset of a uterine contraction. IV oxytocin may be necessary if there is no spontaneous uterine contraction. Threatened preterm delivery may contraindicate use of this test. Aortocaval compression by the pregnant uterus is a known cause of false-positive test. (Ref. 10, pp. 281–283)

72. C. Retroviruses consist of an outer envelope containing a core of single stranded RNA. Human retroviruses were discovered in the late 1970s, and are the cause of adult T-cell leukemia, T-cell variants of hairy cell leukemia, and AIDS. (Ref. 2, pp. 1794–1798)

73. C. With respect to prevention, the risk of developing endocarditis depends on both the type of cardiac condition and on the risk of bacteremia associated with specific procedures. Patients at highest risk for endocarditis include those with prosthetic heart valves, mitral regurgitation, aortic stenosis, and aortic regurgitation. Patients at low risk include those with cardiac pacemakers, atrial septal defects, and coronary artery disease. Procedures with a high risk of bacteremia include dental extractions, urologic procedures, and gastroenterologic and genitourinary surgery; low-risk procedures include gastrointestinal endoscopy, bronchoscopy, intubation of the trachea, and cardiac catheterization. (Ref. 2, pp. 1585, 1588, 1596)

74. A. CEA is a glycoprotein secreted by columnar epithelial cells and may be elevated in a number of malignancies, including colorectal and breast cancer. A variety of benign conditions, including alcoholic cirrhosis, pancreatitis, and emphysema may also result in elevations. Elevated levels of alpha-fetoprotein and/or β-HCG may be found in testicular carcinoma (Ref. 2, pp. 1099, 1100; Ref. 8, p. 377)

75. C. A substitution of valine for glutamic acid at the sixth residue of the beta chain of hemoglobin results in the formation of crescent (sickled) cells, especially during conditions of deoxygenation. While 8% of black Americans are heterozygous for hemoglobins, only 0.15% actually have the disease. A severe hemolytic anemia results but is usually tolerated by the patient. Blood transfusions are usually limited to hypertransfusions at the time of sickle crisis. Sickle crises may present with swollen joints, chest or abdominal pain, or with the central nervous signs listed. Chronic skeletal abnormalities include bone infarcts and aseptic necrosis of the femoral head. Treatment of sickle crises consists of IV fluids, analgesia, and antibiotics if indicated. (Ref. 1, pp. 1519–1522)

76. A. The patient described has changes consistent with acromegaly. Up to 90% of patients with acromegaly have been reported to have an enlarged sella turcica. Impaired glucose tolerance is present in approximately 50%. The release of growth hormone in response to TRH seen in acromegaly is not found in normal patients. (Ref. 1, pp. 1703, 1704)

77. A. The factors and conditions listed, plus other causes of chronic liver disease, appear to predispose to hepatocellular carcinoma. These include $alpha_1$-antitrypsin deficiency, hereditary tyrosinosis, and chronic androgen therapy. Chronic estrogen exposure has been associated with an increased incidence of hepatic adenomas and focal nodular hyperplasia. (Ref. 1, p. 1351)

78. A. The National Cancer Institute recommends annual mammograms for women over 50 years of age and for women ages 35–50 in high-risk groups. High-risk groups include women whose mothers or sisters have had breast cancer, and women with a history of breast cancer. The correct approach to women ages 35–49, not at increased risk, is still undetermined. (Ref. 1, p. 1568)

79. A. These three diagnoses may present with signs and symptoms of Cushing's syndrome and fail to suppress plasma cortisol levels during the overnight dexamethasone suppression test (DST). Patients with depression may fail to suppress their plasma cortisol. However, they do not present clinically with signs of hypercortisolism. (Ref. 1, pp. 1761, 1762)

80. C. Failure to suppress plasma cortisol in response to the high-dose DST is most characteristic of adrenal neoplasms and ectopic ACTH production. Obese patients and patients with pituitary microadenomas characteristically suppress to less than 50% of baseline levels in response to the high-dose dexamethasone suppression test. (Ref. 1, pp. 1761, 1762)

81. B. The normal urinary 17-ketosteroids and abdominal CT scan make an adrenal carcinoma an unlikely cause of this patient's Cushing's syndrome. The ectopic production of ACTH is therefore the most likely source of this patient's hypercortisolism. Anaplastic small cell carcinoma of the lung accounts for the majority of these cases. (Ref. 1, pp. 643, 644)

82. B. Low serum T3 is seen in hypothyroidism, the low-T3 syndrome, and in patients with decreased concentration of thyroxin-binding globulins. Graves' disease is a thyrotoxic state associated with hyperreflexia and an elevated serum T_3. (Ref. 1, p. 1737)

83. C. *Cryptosporidium* and *Isospora* are protozoans that may cause sustained, watery diarrhea in immunocompromised patients. *Shigella* and *Salmonella* cause acute gastrointestinal illnesses. (Ref. 2, pp. 1645, 1646, 1805, 1806)

84. A. Identification of protozoan infections of the gastrointestinal tract is often best accomplished by microscopic examination of a wet preparation of the stool. Cryptosporidiosis, the most common etiology of the above syndrome in a patient at risk for the acquired immunodeficiency syndrome, can also be identified by its characteristic acid-fast positive reaction with either Kinyoun or Ziehl-Neelsen stains. Intestinal biopsy is not felt to be as sensitive as the above measures. Stool culture and sensitivity, while more likely useful in acute-onset diarrhea, would be indicated. (Ref. 2, pp. 1805, 1806, 1882, 1883)

85. B. The reduction of GFR with age is sufficient to decrease the clearance of some drugs, necessitating alterations in their dose. The decline in ventilatory function of the lung with age (decreased vital capacity, forced expiratory volume in one second, and maximal breathing capacity) reduces pulmonary reserve and results in earlier clinical compromise in the presence of superimposed pulmonary disease. There is no large age-related physiologic reduction in hemoglobin; elderly men with hemoglobins less than 13 g/dL and elderly women with hemoglobins less than 12 g/dL should be considered anemic and evaluated appropriately. The fasting blood glucose does not rise significantly with age; fasting blood glucoses between 120 mg% and 140 mg% are in the range of glucose intolerance and those above 140 mg% are in the diabetic range. (Ref. 2, pp. 24, 25; Ref. 21, p. 520)

86. A. These three conditions, plus erosive gastritis, account for almost 90% of upper gastrointestinal hemorrhage. Peptic ulceration, usually in the duodenum, is probably the most common cause. Gastritis, often secondary to drugs (alcohol, nonsteroidal antiinflammatory drugs) or to major trauma, surgery or burns, occurs frequently. Variceal bleeding is most often the result of alcohol cirrhosis in this country. The Mallory-Weiss syndrome is characterized by a mucosal lesion at the esophagogastric junction, preceded by history of retching. Gastric carcinoma is a less common cause of upper gastrointestinal blood loss. (Ref. 1, pp. 180, 181)

87. B. Because their management differs, it is important to distinguish between carotid and vertebrobasilar TIA. Amaurosis fugax (transient unilateral visual loss) is strongly suggestive of carotid

TIA while transient bilateral visual deficits or bilateral motor or sensory deficits suggest vertebrobasilar ischemia. Syncope and vertigo not associated with focal neurologic symptoms and signs are *not* usually manifestations of TIA but are instead caused by other disorders. (Ref. 2, pp. 2168, 2169)

88. A. The primary criteria for brain death include absence of all cerebral and brain stem function for at least 6 hours when the cause of coma is known and depressant drug poisoning is not involved. If the cause of coma is unknown, cerebral and brain stem function must be absent for at least 12 hours, and a negative toxicologic drug screen must be documented. An isoelectric EEG for 30 minutes is a supplementary criterion useful as additional confirmation of brain death when making a decision about organ transplant after 6 hours of absent cerebral and brain stem function. Absence of true spinal reflexes is not required for the diagnosis of brain death. (Ref. 2, pp. 2072, 2073)

89. A. The most common cause of parkinsonism is the idiopathic degeneration of neurons in the substantia nigra and locus ceruleus. Secondary causes of parkinsonism, which may closely resemble idiopathic parkinsonism, include multiple small cerebral (lacunar) infarctions, high dose reserpine and antipsychotic therapy with phenothiazines and butyrophenones, postencephalitic parkinsonism, hypoparathyroidism, and toxic exposures to carbon monoxide and manganese. Bromocriptine is a dopamine receptor agonist used to treat parkinsonism. (Ref. 2, pp. 2143–2145)

90. E. Increased aldosterone secretion in primary aldosteronism results in enhanced urinary potassium excretion in the distal tubule. Similarly, excessive mineralocorticoid secretion as a result of elevated plasma renin activity may accompany salt-wasting renal disease, renal artery stenosis, and Cushing's syndrome. (Ref. 9, pp. 845, 846)

91. A. The patient has reflux esophagitis, which may result in esophageal ulcers and strictures as well as columnarization of the distal esophageal mucosa, normally composed of squamous epithelium. This change in epithelium is termed Barrett's esophagus and is associated with a 10% incidence of subsequent esophageal adenocarcinoma. Achalasia, a disorder associated with a hypertensive lower esophageal sphincter and abnormal peristalsis of the lower two thirds of the esophagus, has no association with reflux esophagitis. (Ref. 1, pp. 1234, 1235)

92. A. The effectiveness of antacids has been verified by endoscopy. More recent therapies have included the H_2 receptor antagonists cimetidine and ranitidine. These agents block the secretion of gastric acid by gastric parietal cells. Sucralfate, an aluminum salt of sulfated sucrose, adheres to granulation tissue and is believed to prevent diffusion of hydrochloric acid to the base of the ulcer. It is as effective as antacids or H_2 receptor antagonists in ulcer therapy. Surgery is generally restricted to patients with disease refractory to medical therapy, perforated or penetrating ulcers, or patients with significant blood loss. (Ref. 1, pp. 1242–1244)

93. A. Migratory arthritis of large peripheral joints may be seen with inflammatory bowel disease, colitis secondary to *Y. enterocolitica*, and Whipple's disease, which is associated with intracellular periodic acid-Schiff-positive bacilliform structures in intestinal mucosa and other tissues. Zollinger-Ellison syndrome (gastric hypersecretion secondary to gastrin-producing tumor resulting in peptic ulcer disease and diarrhea) is not associated with arthritis. (Ref. 1, pp. 617, 1250–1252, 1461, 1462)

94. A. Diabetic gastroparesis is thought to result primarily from autonomic neuropathy; gastric malignancy and anticholinergic medications may delay gastric emptying, while metoclopramide is used to stimulate gastric emptying. (Ref. 1, pp. 369, 1254, 1792)

95. B. Intestinal inflammation should be suspected when large numbers of white blood cells are noted by staining a stool specimen with Wright's or methylene blue stains. Pus is not typically present in the diarrheal stools of patients with giardiasis, irritable bowel syndrome, or viral gastroenteritis. (Ref. 15, pp. 264, 265)

96. B. Tricyclic antidepressants frequently cause orthostatic hypotension, especially in patients with left ventricular dysfunction; the quinidine-like effects of these drugs can result in advanced heart block in patients with baseline cardiac conduction abnormalities and can induce ventricular arrhythmias in some susceptible patients. Prolonged use of benzodiazepines followed by abrupt withdrawal of the drugs can result in a withdrawal syndrome that includes grand mal seizures; a few patients develop paradoxical agitation with benzodiazepines. Lithium may produce reversible hypothyroidism and nephrogenic diabetes insipidus; diuretic therapy may increase serum lithium levels with resultant toxicity. Neuroleptic drugs, for example, phenothiazines and butyrophenones, may cause orthostatic hypotension, obstructive jaundice, and tardive dyskinesia. (Ref. 1, pp. 2100, 2102, 2104)

97. D. Hyperkalemia may produce life-threatening cardiac arrhythmias, including asystole. Asystole is generally preceded by other ECG manifestations of hyperkalemia. In sequential order, these include peaking of T waves, prolongation of the P-R interval, loss of P waves, widening of the QRS complex, and, finally, asystole. An ECG should be obtained emergently to assess the immediate threat of the hyperkalemia to the patient. ECG changes more advanced than peaking of T waves demand immediate therapy to lower the serum potassium level. Serum BUN and creatinine would be important in determining the etiology of the hyperkalemia, but would not change the immediate management of the patient. Serum magnesium and calcium measurements are not emergently needed. (Ref. 2, pp. 548, 549)

98. A. A Life-threatening hyperkalemic cardiotoxicity includes absence of P waves, widening of the QRS complex, and/or ventricular arrhythmias on ECG. Calcium directly counteracts the effects of hyperkalemia on the heart and may be effective within a few minutes; it does not reduce serum potassium concentration and is effective for only 15 to 30 minutes. Glucose, insulin, and sodium bicarbonate drive potassium intracellularly and thereby reduce serum potassium concentration; the onset of action of these agents is within 30 to 60 minutes, and the effect persists for several hours. Oral Kayexalate acts as an exchange resin to remove potassium from the body and reduce serum potassium concentration; its onset of action is delayed several hours and is therefore not useful in the initial treatment of life-threatening hyperkalemia. (Ref. 2, pp. 548, 549)

99. B. The systolic murmur of hypertrophic obstructive cardiomyopathy intensifies upon standing while the systolic murmur of mitral valve prolapse begins earlier in systole and increases in duration; similar changes occur during Valsalva's maneuver. The murmurs of aortic stenosis and mitral regurgitation decrease in intensity with both maneuvers. (Ref. 9, pp. 36, 37)

100. A. Intravenous drug users are at high risk for AIDS. Causes of acute neurologic manifestations in AIDS patients include fungal and protozoan brain infections, tuberculous infections, viral infections, and CNS lymphoma. A CT or MRI scan may be useful in assessing the presence of a localized lesion, as opposed to more diffuse white matter changes. A CSF examination can identify a variety of infections, or other causes of leptomeningeal disease. Primary lymphomas are best diagnosed by stereotactic biopsy. Cerebral angiography is not as sensitive as a MRI or CT scan in identifying intracerebral mass lesions. (Ref. 2, 2204, 2205)

References

1. Petersdorf RG, Adams RD, Braunwald E, et al (eds): *Harrison's Principles of Internal Medicine*, ed 11. New York, McGraw-Hill, 1987.

2. Wyngaarden J, Smith LH, Jr (eds): *Cecil Textbook of Medicine*, ed 18. Philadelphia, WB Saunders, 1988.

3. Wintrobe MM, Lee GR, Boggs DR, et al (eds): *Clinical Hematology*, ed 8. Philadelphia, Lea & Febiger, 1981.

3. Wintrobe MM, Lee GR, Boggs DR, et al (eds): *Clinical Hematology*, ed 8. Philadelphia, Lea & Febiger, 1981.

4. Wilson JD, Foster DW (eds): *Williams Textbook of Endocrinology*, ed 7. Philadelphia, WB Saunders, 1985.

5. Moschella SL, Hurley HJ (eds): *Dermatology*, ed 2. Philadelphia, WB Saunders, 1985.

6. Rubenstein E, Federman DD (eds): *Scientific American Medicine*. New York, Scientific American, 1983.

7. Rudolf AM, Hoffman JIE (eds): *Pediatrics*, ed 18. Norwalk, CT, Appleton and Lange, 1987.

8. DeVita VT, Hellman S, Rosenberg SA (eds): *Cancer, Principles and Practice of Oncology*, ed 2. Philadelphia, JB Lippincott, 1985.

9. Braunwald E (ed): *Heart Disease—A Textbook of Cardiovascular Medicine*, ed 3. Philadelphia, WB Saunders, 1988.

10. Pritchard JA, MacDonald PC, Gant NF (eds): *Williams Obstetrics*, ed 17. Norwalk, CT, Appleton-Century-Crofts, 1985.

11. Hurst JW (ed): *The Heart*, ed 6. New York, McGraw-Hill, 1986.

12. Rodnan GP, Schumacher HR, Zuaifler J (eds): *Primer on the*

Rheumatic Diseases, ed 8. Atlanta, Arthritis Foundation, 1983.

13. Kelley WN, Harris ED Jr, Ruddy S, Sledge CB (eds): *Textbook of Rheumatology*, ed 2. Philadelphia, WB Saunders, 1985.

14. McIntyre KM, Lewis AJ (eds): *Textbook of Advanced Cardiac Life Support*. Dallas, American Heart Association, 1981.

15. Sleisenger MH, Fordtran JS (eds): *Gastrointestinal Disease*, ed 3. Philadelphia, WB Saunders, 1983.

16. Guenter CA, Welch MH (eds): *Pulmonary Medicine*, ed 2. Philadelphia, JB Lippincott, 1982.

17. Goldman DR, Brown FH, Levy WK, Slap GB, Sussman EJ (eds): *Medical Care of the Surgical Patient*. Philadelphia, JB Lippincott, 1982.

18. Sabiston DC Jr (ed): *Textbook of Surgery, The Biological Basis of Surgical Practice*, ed 13. Philadelphia, WB Saunders, 1986.

19. Fishman AD (ed): *Pulmonary Diseases and Disorders*. New York, McGraw-Hill, 1980.

20. Montgomery WH, Donegan J, McIntyre KM (eds): *1985 National Conference on standards and guidelines for cardiopulmonary resuscitation and emergency cardiac care. JAMA* 1986;255:2985–2989.

21. Calkins E, Davis PJ, Ford AB (eds): *The Practice of Geriatrics*. Philadelphia, WB Saunders, 1986.

22. Expert Panel: Report of the National Cholesterol Education Program Expert Panel on detection, evaluation, and treatment of high blood cholesterol in adults. *Arch Intern Med* 1988; 148:36–69.

2

Pictorial

Lee Hixson, MD, John Lederer, MD, and
Barry M. Stults, MD

DIRECTIONS: For each of the questions or incomplete statements below, one or more of the answers or completions given is correct. Select

- **A** if only *1*, *2*, and *3* are correct
- **B** if only *1* and *3* are correct
- **C** if only *2* and *4* are correct
- **D** if only *4* is correct
- **E** if all are correct

Questions 101–103 (refer to Figure 2.1):

101. The differential for the peripheral blood smear in Figure 2.1 includes which of the following?

B

1. Sideroblastic anemias
2. Thalassemia
3. Iron deficiency
4. Autoimmune hemolytic anemia

102. Findings consistent with iron deficiency include

E

1. decreased serum iron
2. thrombocytosis
3. a decreased plasma ferritin
4. an increased serum iron-binding capacity

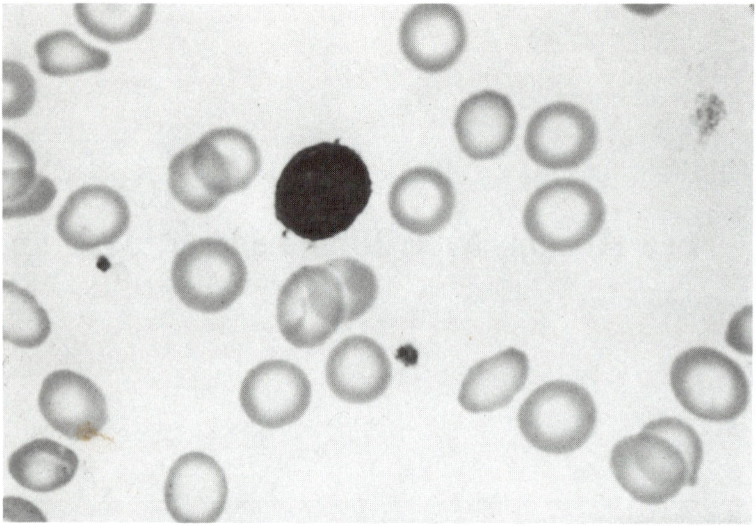

Figure 2.1

Directions Summarized				
A	**B**	**C**	**D**	**E**
1,2,3 only	1,3 only	2,4 only	4 only	all

103. Clinical conditions associated with the peripheral blood depicted in Figure 2.1 include

A

1. GI hemorrhage
2. intestinal malabsorption
3. menstrual blood loss
4. pregnancy

Questions 104–106 (refer to Figure 2.2): A 65-year-old white man presents with complaints of fatigue and lower back pain for 3 months. His hematocrit is noted to be 30 and his peripheral blood is shown in Figure 2.2.

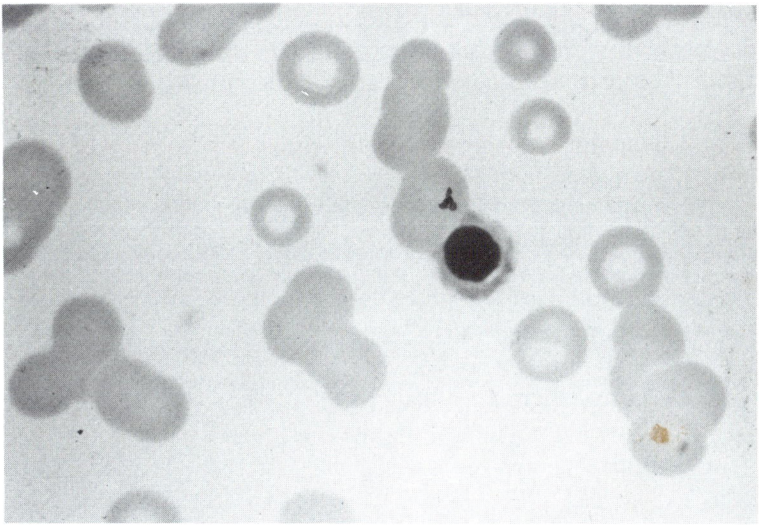

Figure 2.2

104. The abnormalities shown are consistent with
 1. alcoholic liver disease
 2. a myelophthisic process
 3. vitamin B12 deficiency
 4. increased plasma globulins

105. The patient in question 104 develops nausea, vomiting, constipation, and mental confusion. Likely etiologies in this patient include
 1. hyperglycemia
 2. hyperuricemia
 3. hypokalemia
 4. hypercalcemia

106. Treatment for the condition described above might include
 1. IV normal saline
 2. 2–5 U IV insulin/h
 3. 40–100 mg prednisone
 4. allopurinol

Questions 107–109 (refer to Figure 2.3): A 17-year-old Indonesian boy presents with a 2-week history of fevers to 104°F and shaking chills. The peripheral blood smear is shown in Figure 2.3.

107. This abnormality is consistent with
  1. a Döhle body
  2. intravascular *Bartonella bacilliformis*
  3. toxic granulations
  4. *Plasmodium falciparum*

108. Treatment would likely include
  1. high-dose corticosteroids
  2. pyrimethamine-sulfadoxine
  3. broad-spectrum antibiotics
  4. quinine sulfate

Figure 2.3

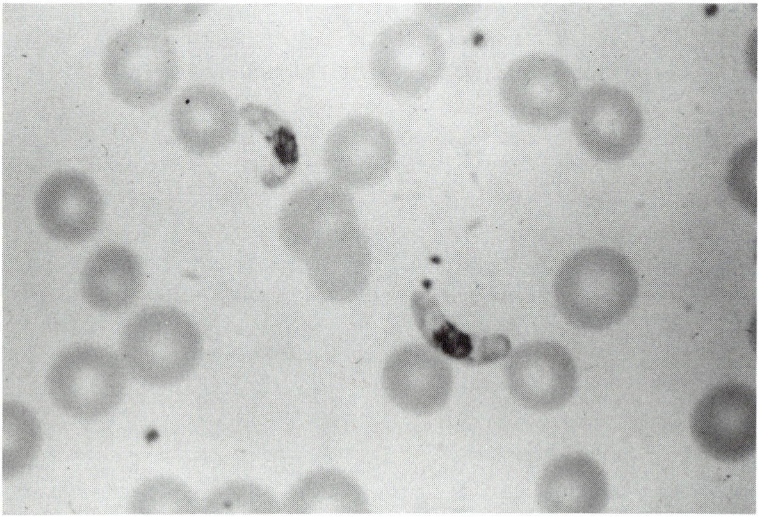

109. Prophylaxis for malaria infections might include
1. weekly po Fansidar
2. judicious use of bed netting and mosquito repellant
3. weekly chemoprophylaxis with 500 mg chloroquine phosphate po
4. avoidance of the tsetse fly Glossina

Questions 110–112 (refer to Figure 2.4):

110. A 58-year-old white man presents with a 2-week history of gingival bleeding. A slide of his peripheral blood is shown in Figure 2.4. Conditions associated with microangiopathic hemolytic anemias and decreased platelet counts (as shown in Figure 2.4) include
1. malignant neoplasm
2. Kasabach-Merritt syndrome
3. sepsis
4. prosthetic valves

Figure 2.4

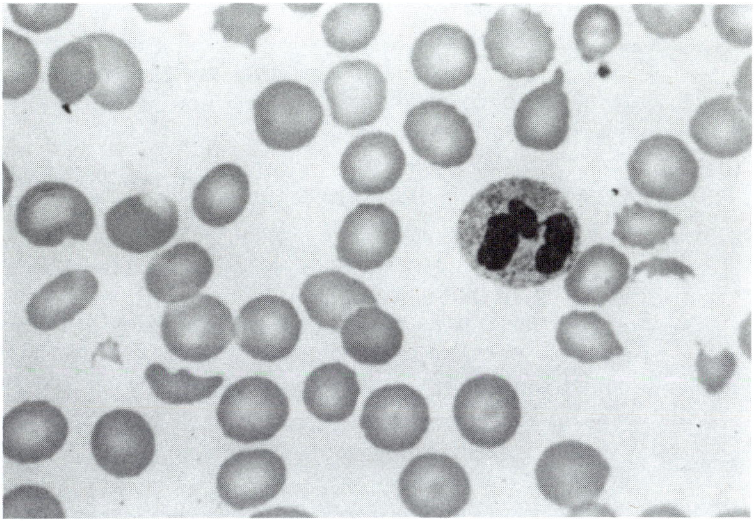

111. Laboratory testing revealed the following values concerning the patient

Prothrombin time 16 sec (normal 10–12 sec)
Plasma fibrinogen 120 mg/dL (normal 160–415 mg/dL)
Hematocrit 33% (normal 45%–55%)
Platelet count 100,000/mm^3 (normal 150,000–400,000/mm^3)

These values are consistent with

1. alcoholic liver disease
2. surreptitious heparin use
3. disseminated intravascular coagulation (DIC)
4. isolated vitamin K deficiency

112. Further examination of the peripheral blood reveals the presence of promyelocytes with hypergranular cytoplasm. Appropriate therapy might include

1. induction therapy for acute promyelocytic leukemia
2. heparin
3. appropriate therapy for infection or acidosis
4. high dose corticosteroids

Questions 113–115 (refer to Figure 2.5):

113. A 30-year-old white male homosexual presents with a 2-month history of fever and weight loss. A biopsy of a skin lesion is interpreted as Kaposi's sarcoma. A diagnosis of acquired immunodeficiency syndrome (AIDS) is made. Other persons at high risk to develop AIDS include

1. IV drug users
2. household contacts of AIDS patients
3. patients with hemophilia A
4. medical personnel exposed to AIDS patients

114. Two months after diagnosis, the patient notes a nonproductive cough and slight dyspnea on exertion. Chest x-ray reveals bilateral interstitial infiltrates. Likely etiologies include

1. pneumococcal pneumonia
2. cytomegalovirus pneumonia
3. disseminated cryptosporidium
4. *Pneumocystis carinii* pneumonia

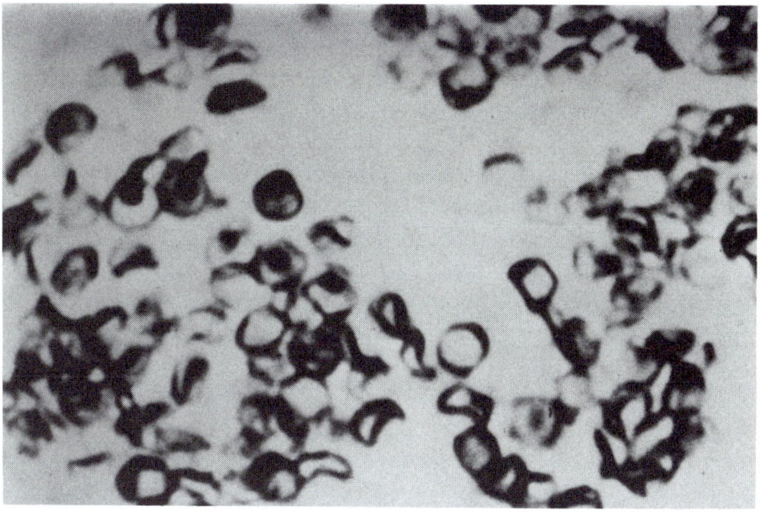

Figure 2.5

115. Due to a failure to respond to broad spectrum antibiotics, the patient underwent open lung biopsy. Staining with Gomori methenamine silver reveals large numbers of the organisms shown in Figure 2.5. Treatment options include

1. IV erythromycin
2. parenteral pentamidine
3. IV acyclovir
C **4.** oral trimethoprim-sulfamethoxazole

Questions 116–120 (refer to Figure 2.6):

116. A 27-year-old sexually active white man presents with a 1-day history of fever and right Achilles tendon pain. A purpuric skin lesion, seen in Figure 2.6, is present on the dorsum of his right hand. Diagnosis of this patient's illness often can be established by

1. culturing scrapings of the skin lesion
2. culturing the blood
3. right ankle joint aspiration and culture of the joint fluid
4. direct fluorescent antibody staining of skin lesion scrapings

117. Despite attempts to identify the etiology of the patient's illness, no diagnosis is made. Eight days after onset of his symptoms, the patient notes a tender, erythematous swelling of his left knee. Which of the following would be useful in diagnosing his condition?

1. Aspiration of the left knee and culture of the joint fluid
2. Pharyngeal culture
3. Rectal culture
4. Blood cultures

Figure 2.6

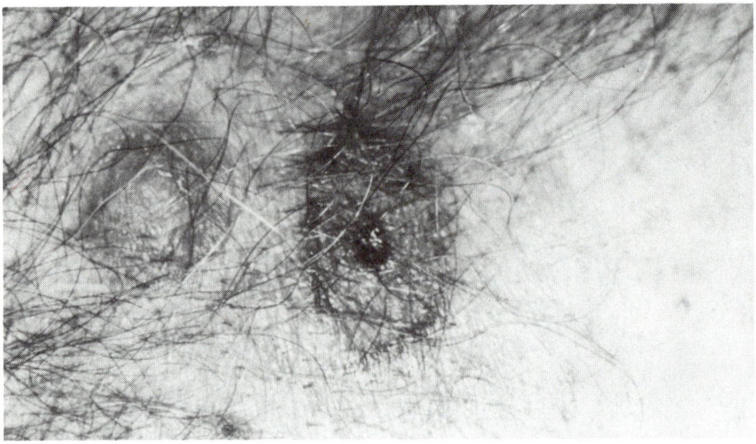

118. A Gram's-stained slide obtained from the patient's anal canal reveals intracellular Gram-negative diplococci. Laboratory techniques that would help identify this agent as *N. gonorrhoeae* include

1. a growth on Thayer-Martin agar
2. a positive oxidase test
3. the ability to metabolize glucose
4. the ability to metabolize maltose

119. Recommended therapy for disseminated gonococcemia includes

1. aqueous penicillin G 10 million U/day IV for a minimum of 3 days, followed by ampicillin 500 mg 4 times a day po for 10 days
2. 4.8 million U aqueous procaine penicillin given in two sites IM, plus 1 g probenecid po
3. ampicillin 3.5 g po, with 1 g probenecid, followed by ampicillin 500 mg po for 10 days
4. tetracycline 500 mg 4 times a day for 7 days

120. Female sexual contacts of the above patient who have contracted gonorrhea

1. have approximately a 15% risk of developing pelvic inflammatory disease (PID)
2. are often asymptomatic or minimally symptomatic
3. may have as high as a 50% incidence of infertility after recurrent PID
4. may present with the clinical picture of cystitis

Questions 121–123 (refer to Figure 2.7):

121. A 55-year-old black man presents with a 2-month history of fatigue. His hematocrit is 34%. A smear of his peripheral blood is shown in Figure 2.7. These changes are consistent with

1. chronic blood loss and iron deficiency
2. vitamin B12 deficiency
3. sickle cell anemia
4. folate deficiency

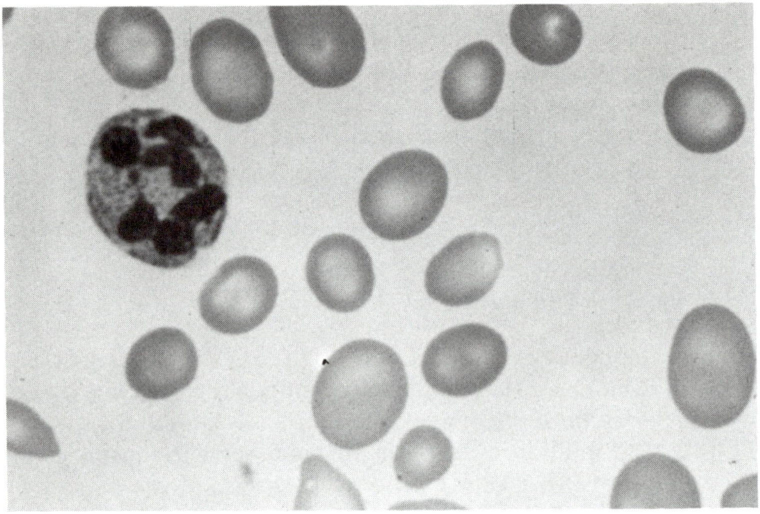

Figure 2.7

122. Further evaluation of this patient would likely include
   1. serum B12 levels
   2. stool guaiacs
   3. serum or red blood cell folate levels
   4. hemoglobin electrophoresis

123. Vitamin B12 absorption
   1. requires the presence of intrinsic factor
   2. may be decreased in patients with regional enteritis
   3. may be assessed by a Schilling test
   4. occurs primarily in the duodenum

Questions 124–126 (refer to Figure 2.8):

124. A 55-year-old white woman presents with a 2-month history of weakness. Her hematocrit is 30%. The peripheral blood smear revealed the abnormality shown in Figure 2.8. Possible diagnoses would include

1. acute lymphoblastic leukemia
2. chronic granulocytic leukemia in blast crisis
3. chronic lymphocytic leukemia
4. acute granulocytic leukemia

125. Bone marrow aspiration and biopsy are performed. Differential count of the marrow reveals greater than 50% of the cells to be blasts. The blasts would characteristically

1. stain positively for Sudan B black
2. contain the Philadelphia chromosome
3. stain positively for myeloperoxidase
4. have elevated terminal deoxynucleotidyl transferase levels

Figure 2.8

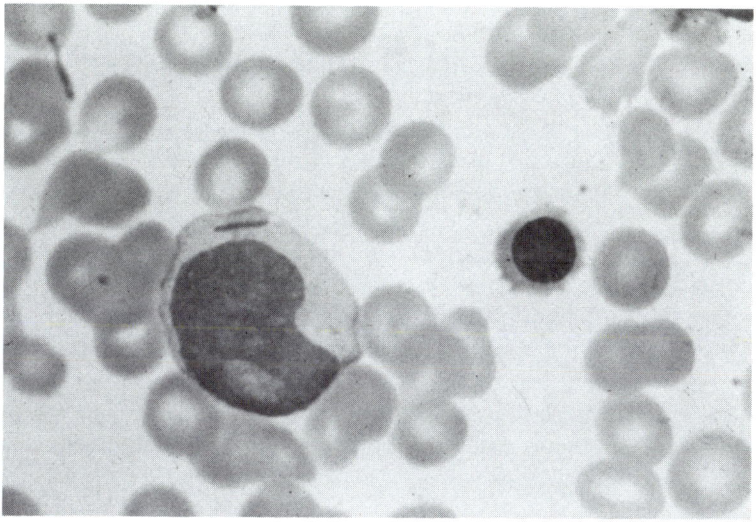

126. Poor prognostic factors in patients with acute myelogenous leukemia include
1. an age of greater than 70 years
A **2.** chromosomal abnormalities t(8;21), t(15;17)
3. a history of preleukemia
4. the presence of increased numbers of hypergranular promyelocytes

Questions 127–129 (refer to Figure 2.9):

127. A 40-year-old man with a 6-year history of intermittent bloody diarrhea undergoes the barium enema shown in Figure 2.9. GI complications of this disease include
1. toxic megacolon
B **2.** aphthous ulcers
3. colon carcinoma
4. anal fistula

128. Which of the following statements pertaining to this disease are true?
1. Prophylactic colectomy is recommended in patients with universal colon involvement for longer than 5 years
A **2.** Ten percent of patients after the first attack will have a prolonged remission
3. Anticholinergic drugs and opiates are generally effective in controlling the diarrhea
4. The appearance of the colonic mucosa in this disease may be mimicked by acute infectious colitis secondary to *Salmonella, Shigella, Campylobacter,* and amebiasis

129. Articular manifestations of inflammatory bowel disease (IBD)
1. occur in approximately 25% of patients with IBD
2. are often monoarticular or polyarticular involving peripheral joints
A **3.** can present as ankylosing spondylitis
4. always correlate with the activity of the underlying bowel disease

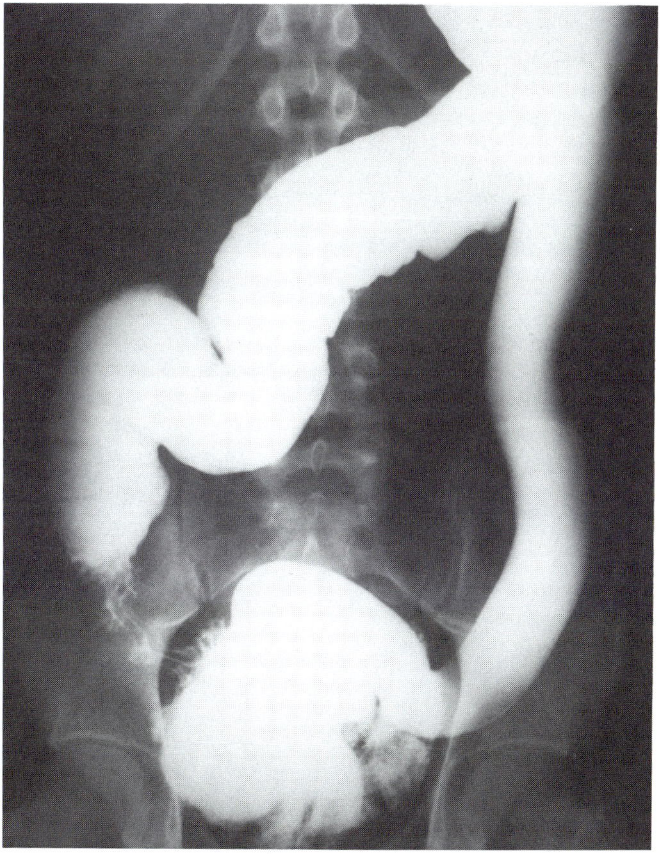

Figure 2.9

Questions 130–132 (refer to Figure 2.10):

130. The patient develops a small ulcer just superior to his right lateral malleolus, and the ulcer grows rapidly in size and depth to the extent shown in Figure 2.10. Appropriate therapy of the ulcer would include

1. wide excision and debridement with grafting
2. high-dose IV penicillin
3. ketoconazole
4. topical and systemic corticosteroids

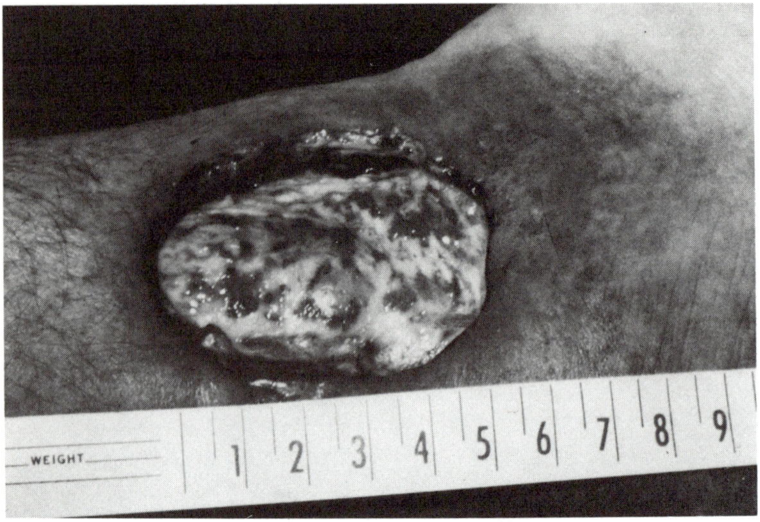

Figure 2.10

131. Prior to treatment with methylprednisolone therapy, an intermediate strength 5 TU PPD is placed, which results in 15 mm of induration 48 hours later. The patient is unaware of any past exposure to tuberculosis and his chest radiograph is normal. Appropriate subsequent actions would include
1. annual PPD (purified protein derivative)
2. serial chest radiograph every 6 months for 2 years
3. rifampin 600 mg po qd for 6 months
4. isoniazid 300 mg po qd for 12 months

132. Major toxicity associated with the use of isoniazid includes
1. hepatitis
2. influenza-like syndrome
3. peripheral neuropathy
4. thrombocytopenia

Questions 133–135 (refer to Figure 2.11):

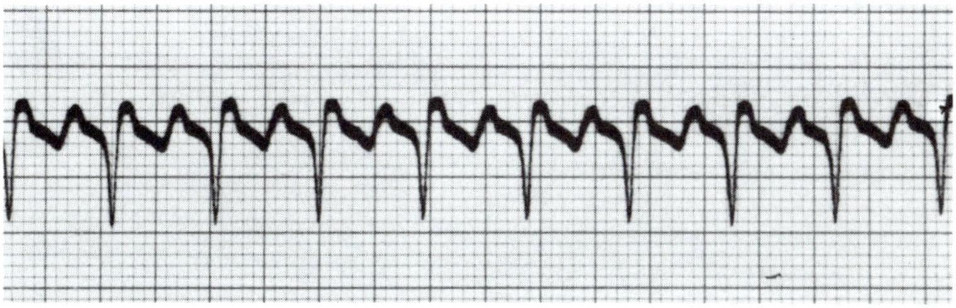

Figure 2.11

133. The rhythm in Figure 2.11 may be associated with which of the following?

1. Rheumatic heart disease
2. Dilated cardiomyopathy
3. Pericarditis
4. Quinidine toxicity

134. Which of the following statements concerning this rhythm are true?

1. Sinus rhythm is usually restored by carotid sinus massage
2. The incidence of systemic emboli is less than that associated with atrial fibrillation
3. DC cardioversion employing >200 joules is generally needed for conversion to sinus rhythm
4. The ventricular rate may increase after administration of quinidine, disopyramide, or procainamide

135. DC cardioversion may be complicated by which of the following?

1. Ventricular fibrillation
2. Systemic emboli
3. ST-segment elevation with elevations of myocardial enzymes
4. Pericarditis

Questions 136–138 (refer to Figure 2.12):

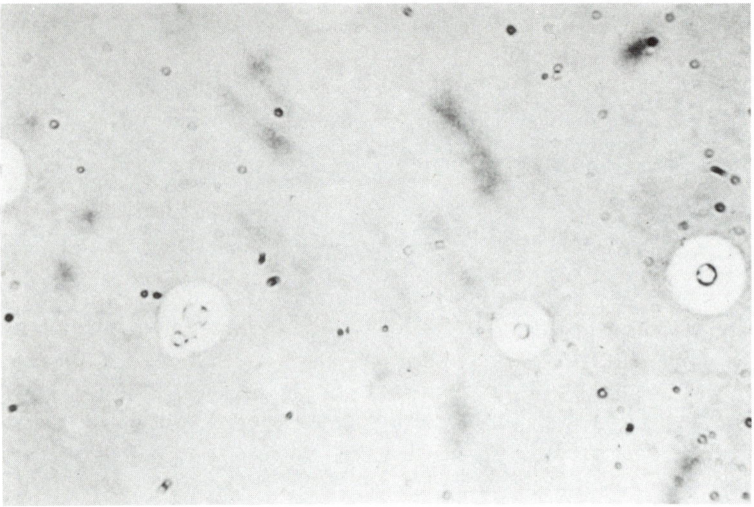

Figure 2.12

136. A 40-year-old white man with diffuse histiocytic lymphoma develops nausea, headache, and blurred vision. Lumbar puncture reveals CSF with

Protein 85 mg/100 mL (normal < 40 mg/100 mL)
Glucose 35 mg/100 mL: serum glucose 130 mg/100 mL (normal CSF glucose: serum glucose ratio > 60%)
Leukocytes 80 cells/mm^3: 86% lymphocytes, 15% neutrophils (normal < 5 cells/mm^3 with 100% lymphocytes)
Red blood cells 0

The most likely diagnoses are

1. tuberculous meningitis
2. pneumococcal meningitis
3. fungal meningitis
4. subarachnoid hemorrhage

137. Examination of the spinal fluid of this patient reveals the abnormality seen in Figure 2.12. Other studies likely to diagnose this condition include

1. CT scan of the brain
2. blood culture
3. technetium brain scan
4. latex agglutination cryptococcal antigen of CSF or serum

138. Complications commonly associated with therapy include

1. hypokalemia
2. colitis
3. renal insufficiency
4. peripheral neuropathy

Questions 139–141 (refer to Figure 2.13):

Figure 2.13

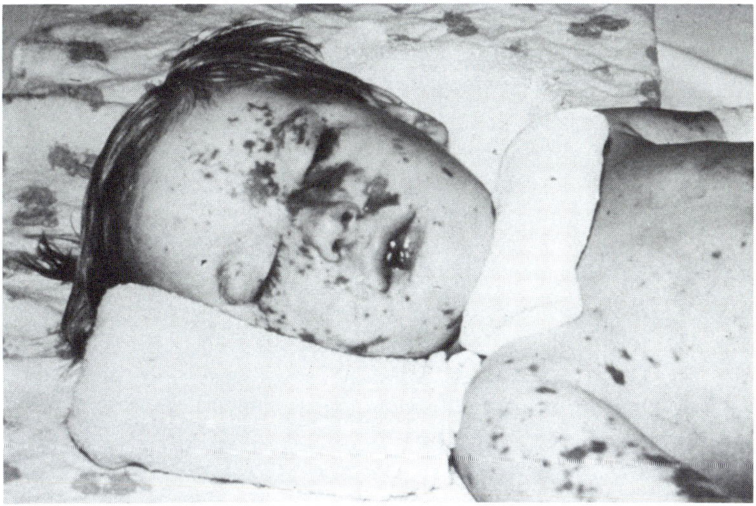

139. A 3-year-old boy presents with a several-hour history of fever, altered mental status, and the rash shown in Figure 2.13. The differential diagnosis would include

1. hypersensitivity vasculitis
2. meningococcemia with meningitis
3. enteroviral infection
4. pneumococcal sepsis

140. The diagnosis of meningococcal disease may be established by

1. spinal fluid culture
2. culture of petechial scrapings
3. counterimmunoelectrophoresis
4. culture of the nasopharynx

141. Prophylaxis for meningococcal disease

1. should be given to all intimate contacts
2. can be achieved by rifampin 600 mg/day for 2 days
3. can be achieved by minocycline 100 mg every 12 hours for 5 days
4. can be achieved by penicillin VK 500 mg every 12 hours for 5 days

Questions 142–143 (refer to Figure 2.14):

142. Patients with the disorder manifested by the hands appearing in Figure 2.14 commonly demonstrate which of the following?

1. Subcutaneous nodules on the extensor surfaces of the forearms in 20%–25% of patients
2. Positive serum rheumatoid factor in 70% of patients
3. Reduction in hemolytic complement levels in joint fluid to less than one third of serum levels
4. Normal erythrocyte sedimentation rate (ESR) in most patients

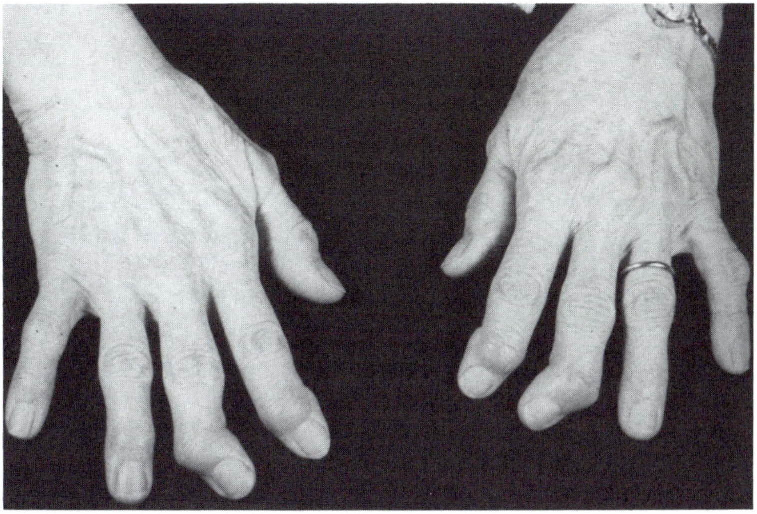

Figure 2.14

143. Symptomatic patients with the disorder shown in Figure 2.14 may derive therapeutic benefit from

1. aspirin or nonsteroidal antiinflammatory agents

2. oral corticosteroids when symptoms are severe

3. isometric exercises with the affected joints maintained at rest

4. isotonic exercises involving affected joints, moving them through a full range of motion against progressively increasing resistance

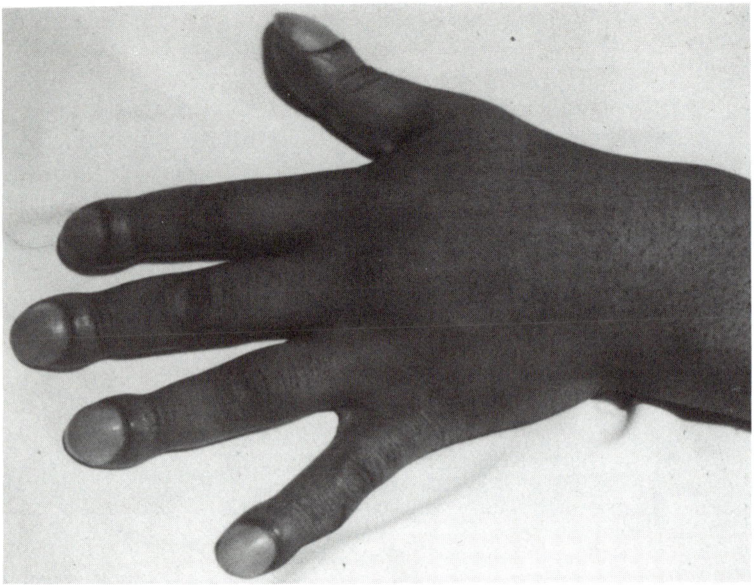

Figure 2.15

Questions 144–145 (refer to Figure 2.15):

144. The abnormality in Figure 2.15 is commonly associated with which of the following disorders?
1. Bronchogenic carcinoma
2. Bronchiectasis
3. Cyanotic congenital heart disease
4. Regional enteritis

145. Hypertrophic osteoarthropathy may accompany the abnormality in Figure 2.15. This syndrome is characterized by

1. pain and tenderness in the distal upper and lower extremities
2. morning stiffness and polyarthritis involving the knees, ankles, wrists, elbows, and metacarpophalangeal joints
3. periosteal new bone formation in radiographs of distal parts of long bones
4. frequent presence of subcutaneous nodules on the extensor surface of the forearm

Questions 146–147 (refer to Figure 2.16):

Figure 2.16

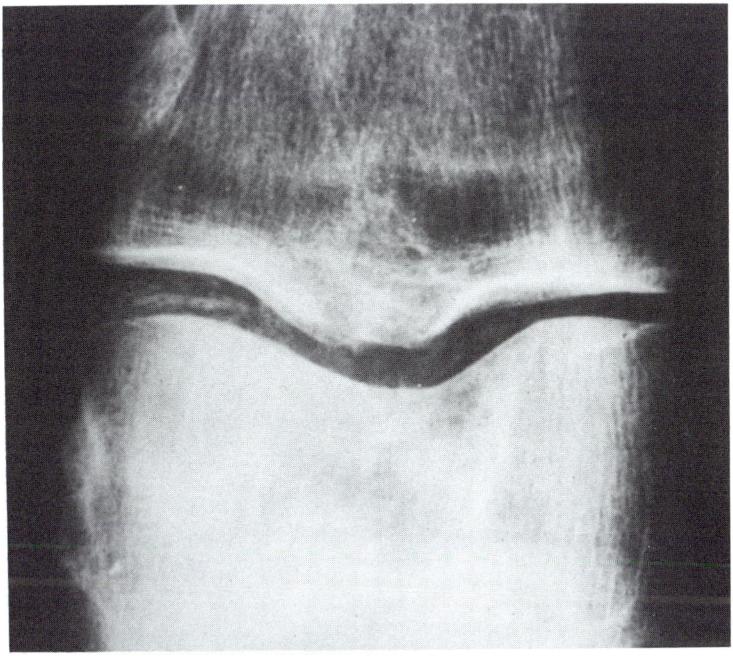

146. Patients with the radiographic findings in Figure 2.16 may present with which of the following clinical syndromes?

1. Acute monoarticular arthritis involving the knee, ankle, wrist, or elbow
2. Progressive symmetrical degenerative changes in multiple joints (knees, wrists, metacarpophalangeal joints, hips, shoulders) with joint space narrowing
3. Symmetrical inflammatory changes (morning stiffness, synovial thickening) of knees, wrists, and metatarsophalangeal joints
4. Absence of joint symptoms

147. Aspirated joint fluid from the knee joint seen in Figure 2.16 characteristically will demonstrate

1. positive bacterial culture
2. microscopic, needle-shaped crystals that have strongly negative birefringence under polarized light
3. glucose concentration less than 25% of a simultaneously measured serum glucose level
4. rod- or rhomboid-shaped crystals that have weakly positive birefringence under polarized light

Questions 148–150 (refer to Figure 2.17):

148. The differential diagnosis of the abnormality in Figure 2.17 includes

1. cellulitis and/or septic arthritis
2. calcium pyrophosphate deposition disease
3. gout
4. Reiter's syndrome

149. Initial therapy for an acute attack of gouty arthritis should include which of the following?

1. Probenecid
2. Allopurinol
3. Low purine diet
4. Colchicine or a nonsteroidal antiinflammatory agent

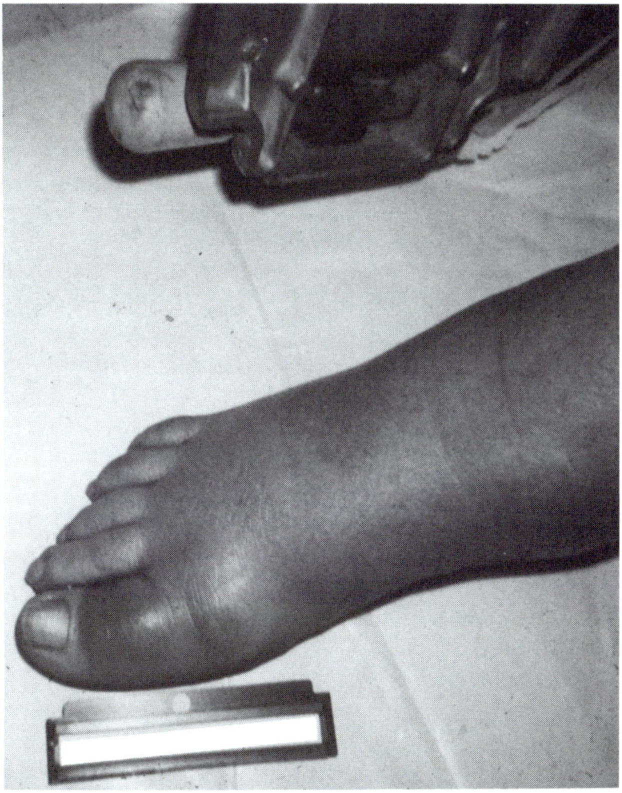

Figure 2.17

150. A diagnosis of acute gouty arthritis may be established by which of the following?
   1. Hyperuricemia
   2. Inflammatory involvement of the metatarsophalangeal joint of the great toe (podagra)
   3. Improvement in symptoms and signs with colchicine therapy
   4. Intraleukocytic sodium urate crystals in aspirated joint fluid

Questions 151–152 (refer to Figure 2.18):

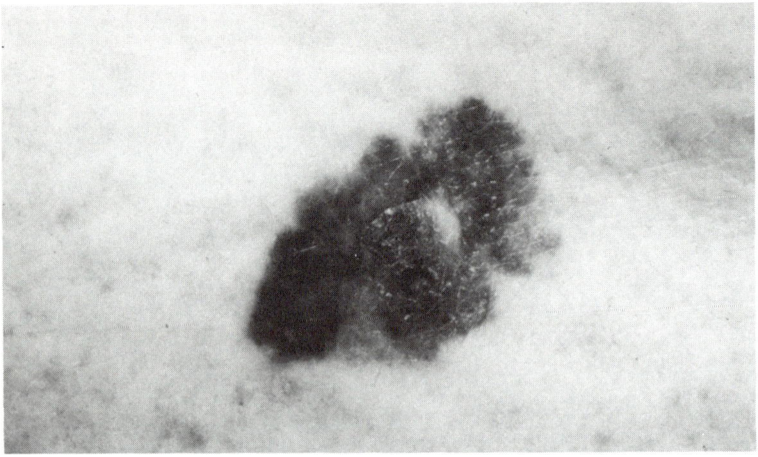

Figure 2.18

151. Characteristics of the skin lesion shown in Figure 2.18 that are suggestive of malignancy include
  1. black color
  2. irregular border
  3. nonraised
  4. multiple shades of color

152. Studies have associated which of the following with an increased risk of melanoma?
  1. Increased latitude
  2. Persons who tan poorly
  3. History of excessive tanning
  4. The presence of large, congenital melanocytic nevi

Questions 153–156 (refer to Figure 2.19):

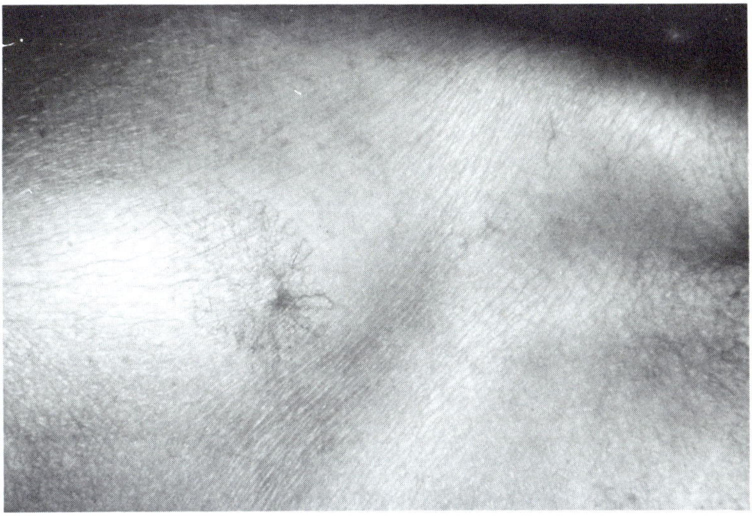

Figure 2.19

153. A 30-year-old man presents with abdominal distention and the cutaneous abnormality adjacent to the axilla shown in Figure 2.19. Other associated findings on physical exam that might be expected include

1. gynecomastia
2. testicular length less than 3 cm
3. palmar erythema
4. hirsutism

154. The patient undergoes a liver biopsy that reveals postnecrotic cirrhosis. Which virus(es) could be responsible for this process?

1. Hepatitis A
2. Non-A, non-B hepatitis
3. Cytomegalovirus (CMV)
4. Hepatitis B

155. Factors that might precipitate portal systemic encephalopathy (PSE) in this patient include
  1. GI bleeding
  2. high carbohydrate diet
  3. hypokalemic alkalosis
  4. vitamin K administration

156. Treatment of PSE would include
  1. restriction or elimination of dietary protein
  2. neomycin 500 mg q 6 hours orally
  3. lactulose orally until diarrhea occurs and then to maintain 2–4 loose stools/day
  4. sedation with a benzodiazepine

Questions 157–158 (refer to Figure 2.20):

Figure 2.20

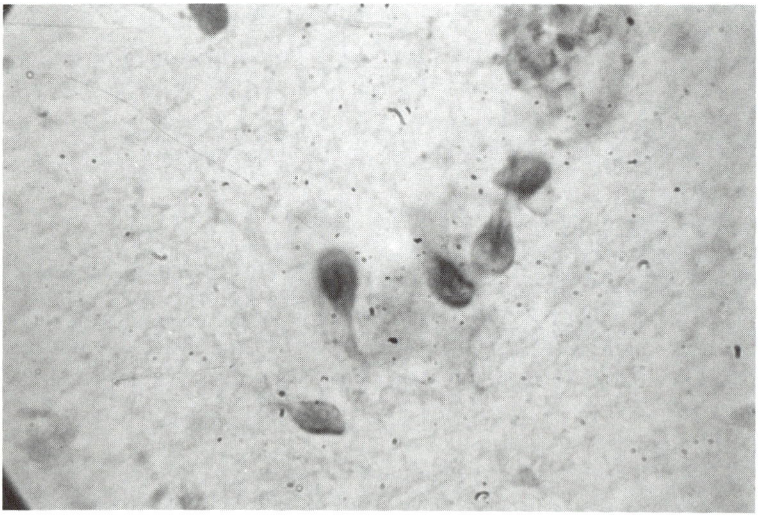

157. Which statement(s) concerning the organism apparent in the microscopic stool smear shown in Figure 2.20 is (are) true?
1. It is transmitted by snails
2. It is the most frequently identified intestinal parasite in the United States
3. It is responsible for typhoid fever
4. It is common in homosexuals

158. Laboratory findings that may accompany infection with this agent include
1. IgA deficiency
2. fecal leukocytes
3. steatorrhea
4. peripheral eosinophilia

Questions 159–160 (refer to Figure 2.21):

Figure 2.21

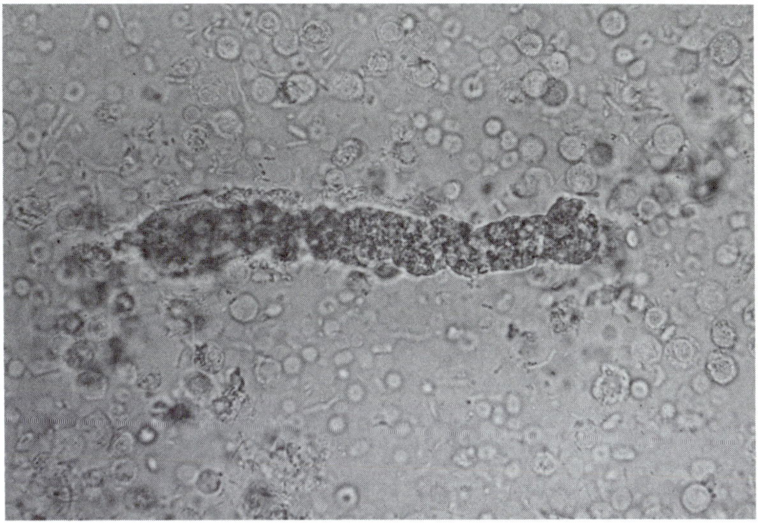

159. A 30-year-old man acutely develops dark "smoky-appearing urine," mild edema of the hands, feet, and periorbital region of the face, and is found to have a blood pressure of 150/100. Urinalysis reveals a specific gravity of 1.020, 3+ protein, 80–100 RBCs/high power field, no WBCs, and many of the structures seen in Figure 2.21. Serum chemistries reveal creatinine = 1.8 mg/dL (normal range = 0.6–1.2 mg/dL), uric acid = 11.1 mg/dL (normal range = 3.5–7.2 mg/dL). Differential diagnosis of this clinical syndrome includes

B

1. membranous nephropathy and minimal change nephrotic syndrome (MCNS)
2. poststreptococcal glomerulonephritis, IgA nephropathy, and antiglomerular basement membrane glomerulonephritis
3. obstructive uropathy from uric acid calculi
4. subacute bacterial endocarditis, visceral pyogenic abscess

160. Useful diagnostic tests to confirm the etiology of this young man's illness would include

A

1. antistreptolysin O (ASO) titer or streptozyme test (detects antibody to five streptococcal antigens in a single test)
2. serum levels of complement components C_3 and C_4
3. antiglomerular basement membrane (anti-GBM) antibody
4. blood cultures

Questions 161–162 (refer to Figure 2.22):

161. The abnormality in Figure 2.22 is commonly associated with which of the following?

K

1. Anterior flexion of the lumbar and thoracic spine
2. Acute anterior uveitis
3. Increased prevalence of the HLA-B27 histocompatibility antigen
4. Peripheral arthritis involving the hips and shoulders

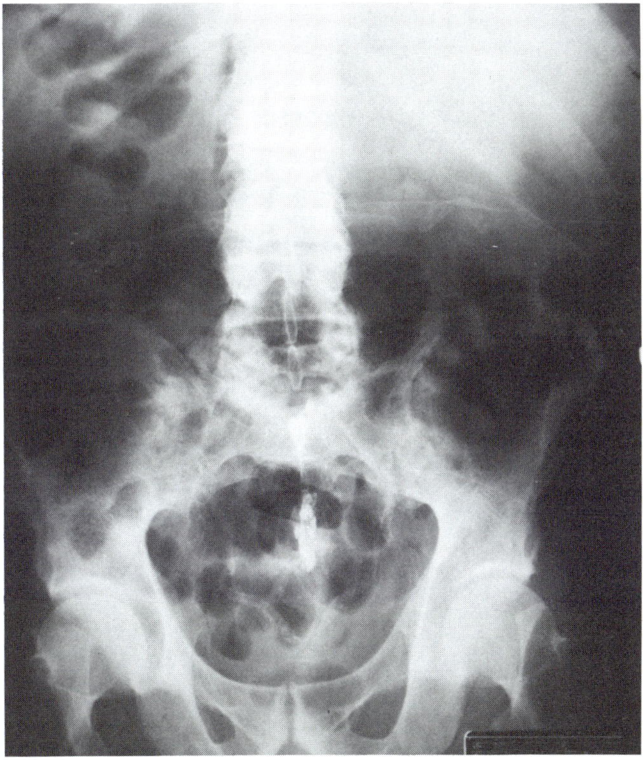

Figure 2.22

162. Therapy for the disorder seen in Figure 2.22 should generally include

1. corticosteroid therapy to halt progression of the disease
2. indomethacin or one of the newer nonsteroidal antiinflammatory agents to control pain
3. gold therapy to minimize the dose of corticosteroids required to halt progression of the disease
4. postural adjustments using physical therapy and exercise programs

Questions 163–165 (refer to Figure 2.23): A 52-year-old man presents with a 1-month history of cough productive of green and brown sputum, daily fever, night sweats, anorexia, and a 15-pound weight loss. His chest radiograph is seen in Figure 2.23.

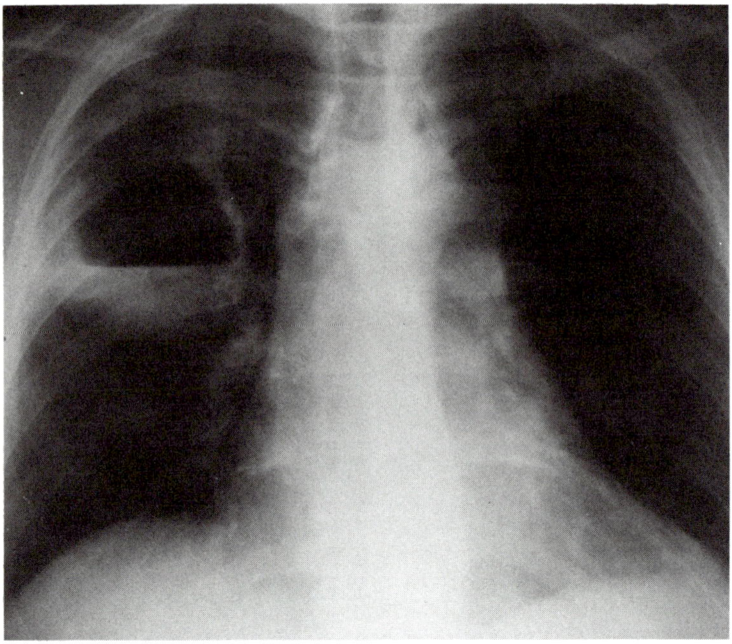

Figure 2.23

163. Additional clinical data potentially pertinent to the etiology of the lesion in Figure 2.23 include

1. presence of dysphagia
2. history of surgery under general anesthesia within the past 3 months
3. history of alcoholism or narcotic addiction
4. severe gingivitis on physical examination

164. Differential diagnosis of the lesion in Figure 2.23 commonly includes

1. tuberculosis
2. bronchogenic carcinoma
3. anaerobic infection
4. pneumococcal infection

165. Cultures of a transtracheal aspirate obtained from this patient reveal *Fusobacterium nucleatum*, *Peptostreptococcus*, anaerobic streptococci, and *Bacteroides melaninogenicus*. Antibiotics that would generally be effective therapy for this patient include

1. penicillin
2. clindamycin
3. penicillin and metronidazole
4. gentamicin

DIRECTIONS: Each of the questions or incomplete statements below is followed by suggested answers or completions. Select the one that is best in each case.

Questions 166–169 (refer to Figure 2.24):

166. A 70-year-old man with a history of hypertension presents with acute confusion, mild hypotension, and tachypnea of 2-hour duration. His chest radiograph reveals pulmonary vascular redistribution with a normal size heart. His ECG is shown in Figure 2.24. The most likely diagnosis is

A. pulmonary embolus
B. acute myocarditis
C. pericarditis with tamponade
D **D.** myocardial infarction
E. dissection of the descending aorta

167. ST-segment elevation may be secondary to all of the following except

A. ventricular aneurysm
B. myocardial infarction
C **C.** coronary artery spasm
D. pericarditis
E. pulmonary embolus

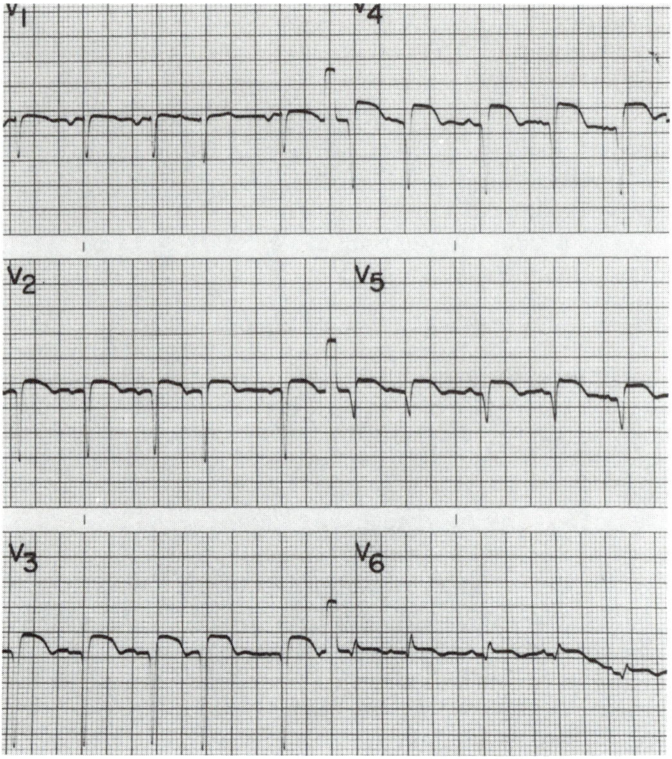

Figure 2.24

168. The patient is at increased risk to develop all of the following except

A. complete atrioventricular (AV) block
B. mitral regurgitation
C. pericarditis
D. mural thrombus
E. endocarditis

169. The patient's blood pressure falls to 70/40 and he becomes more confused. He now demonstrates bilateral crackles one-half way up both lung fields. The most appropriate initial intervention would be

A. IV bolus of 1 L normal saline
B. pulmonary artery catheter placement to measure pulmonary wedge pressure
C. rapid digitalization and IV furosemide
D. dopamine drip at 10 μg/kg/min
E. pericardiocentesis

Question 170 (refer to Figure 2.25):

170. The patient suddenly loses consciousness and his monitored rhythm is demonstrated in Figure 2.25. The appropriate immediate response would be

A. IV bolus of lidocaine 100 mg
B. initiate closed-chest compression
C. IV bolus of 50 mEq $NaHCO_3$
D. DC cardioversion with 200 joules
E. IV bolus of bretylium, 350 mg

Figure 2.25

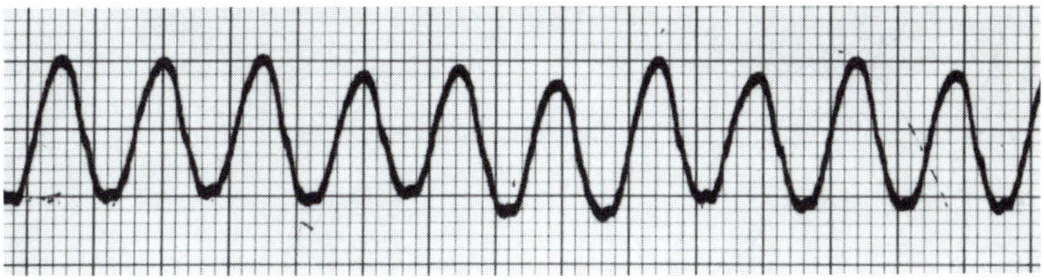

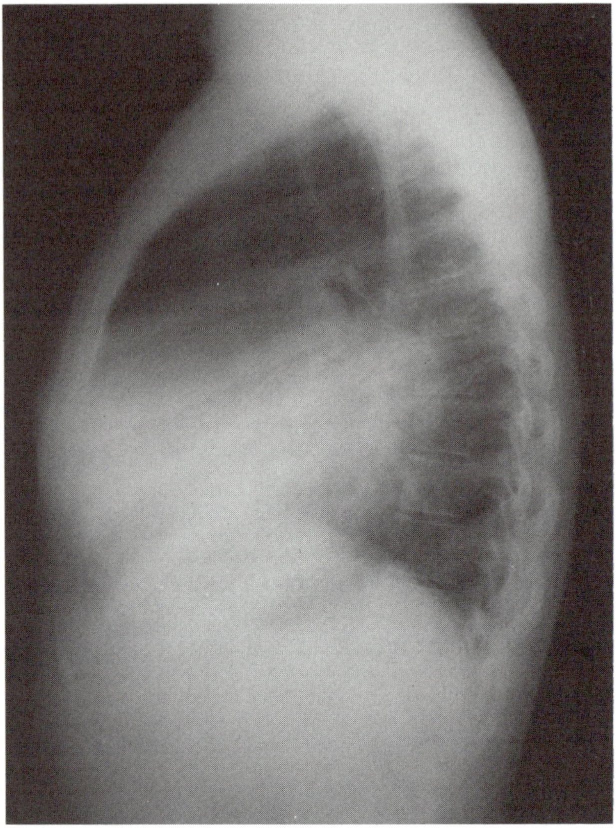

Figure 2.26

Questions 171–172 (refer to Figures 2.26–2.28):

171. A 60-year-old man presents with dyspnea on exertion; his chest radiograph and ECG rhythm are shown in Figures 2.26–2.28. The most likely etiology for the rhythm abnormality is

- **A.** coronary artery disease
- **B.** hyperthyroidism
- **C.** sick sinus syndrome
- **D.** mitral valve disease
- **E.** pulmonary embolus

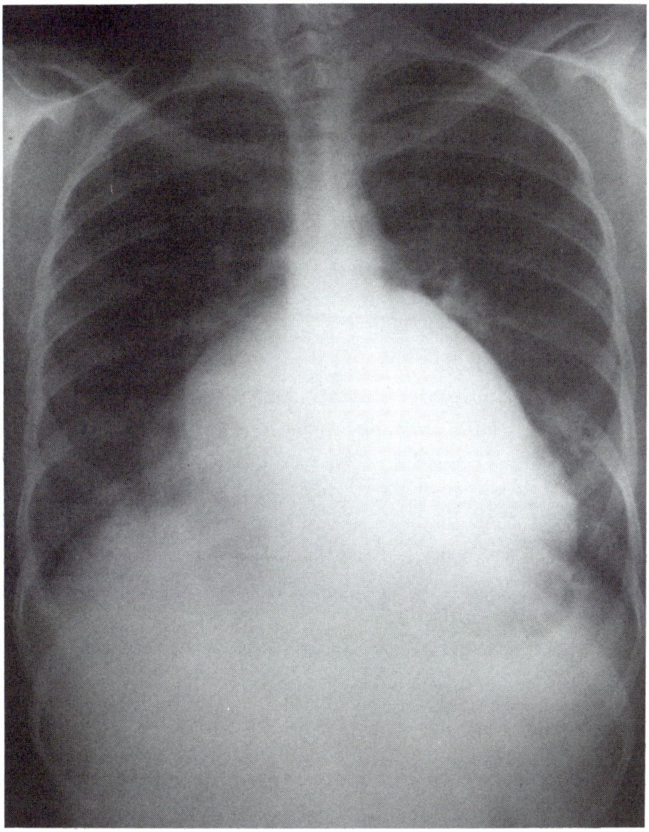

Figure 2.27

172. Appropriate therapy at the time of presentation would include

A **A.** anticoagulation and digitalization
B. propranolol
C. lidocaine
D. DC cardioversion
E. bretylium

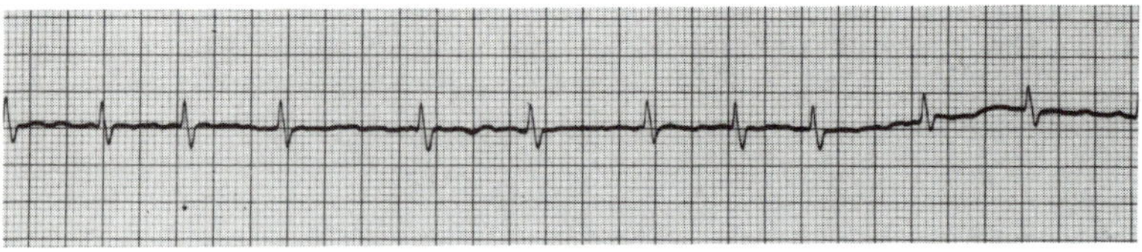

Figure 2.28

Questions 173–175 (refer to Figure 2.29):

173. After loading with digoxin, the patient's ventricular rate slows to 80, but he remains in the same rhythm. Following 3 weeks of oral anticoagulation, quinidine is added to the same daily dose of digoxin to attempt pharmacologic cardioversion; 48 hours later the ECG shown in Figure 2.29 is obtained. The rhythm in Figure 2.29 suggests

A. hypocalcemia
B. hypercalcemia
C. digoxin toxicity
D. hypokalemia
E. hypomagnesemia

Figure 2.29

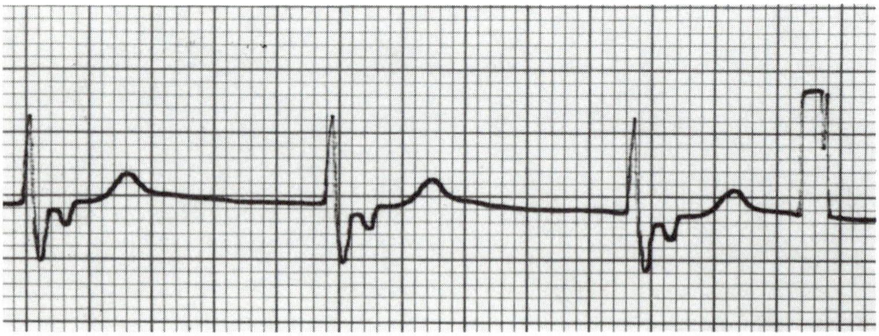

174. Digoxin cardiac toxicity may be facilitated or precipitated by all of the following except

A. hypokalemia, hypomagnesemia, and hypercalcemia
B. concurrent therapy with verapamil or amiodarone
C. concurrent therapy with cholestyramine, neomycin, or nifedipine
D. concurrent pulmonary disease with hypoxemia, hypercapnia, and cor pulmonale
E. increasing severity of heart disease

175. Potentially useful treatments for serious arrhythmias due to digitalis intoxication include all those listed below except

A. quinidine or procainamide for serious ventricular and supraventricular tachyarrhythmias
B. potassium for supraventricular and ventricular tachyarrhythmias
C. lidocaine and phenytoin for serious ventricular and supraventricular tachyarrhythmias
D. atropine or electrical pacing for symptomatic bradyarrhythmias
E. digoxin-specific antibodies

Questions 176–177 (refer to Figure 2.30):

176. The gross pathologic specimen from a 27-year-old patient who undergoes a colectomy is shown in Figure 2.30. Histologic examination reveals multiple areas with adenomatous changes. The most likely diagnosis is

A. Peutz-Jeghers syndrome
B. familial polyposis coli
C. juvenile polyposis
D. Cowden's syndrome
E. pneumatosis cystoides intestinalis

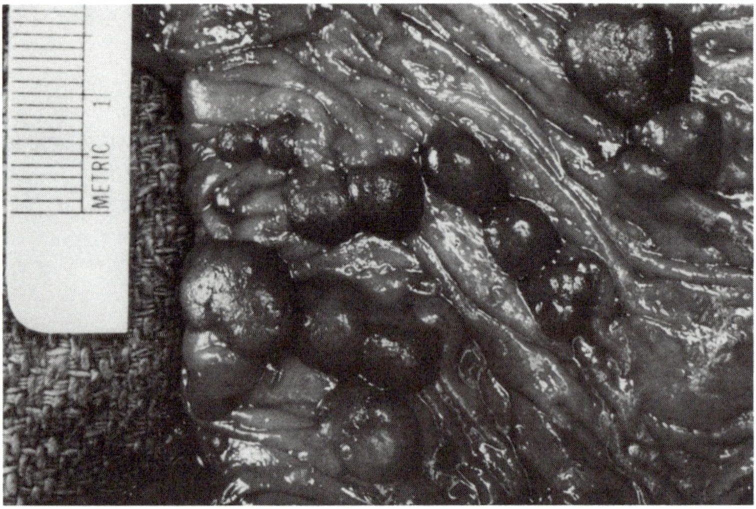

Figure 2.30

177. The patient was initially referred to a physician because the same abnormality was found previously in an older sibling. Prior to surgery, the patient had colonoscopy, which revealed multiple polyps throughout the colon and rectum. His physician recommended total proctocolectomy with ileostomy because

A. this syndrome frequently evolves into ulcerative colitis
B. the patient is at high risk for recurrent bowel obstruction and/or intussusception
C. prophylactic colectomy will protect against the subsequent development of associated liver disease
D. the development of colon cancer is inevitable
E. recurrent life-threatening GI hemorrhage characterizes this syndrome

Questions 178–180 (refer to Figure 2.31):

178. Etiologies of the radiographic abnormality seen in Figure 2.31 include

A. chronic alcohol abuse
B. islet-cell tumors
C. hyperparathyroidism
D. severe protein calorie malnutrition
E. all of the above

Figure 2.31

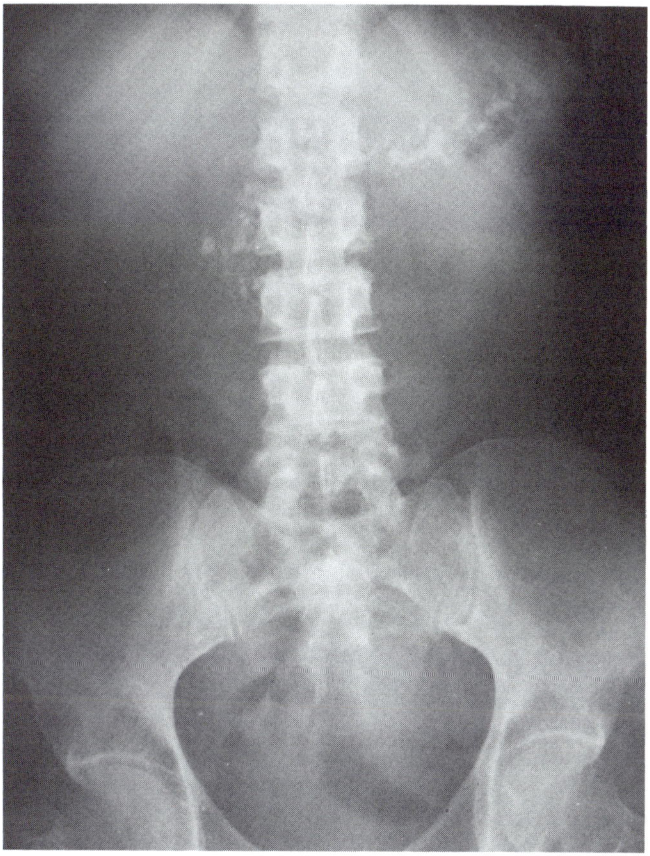

179. Common laboratory findings associated with this entity include
- **A.** steatorrhea
- **B.** macrocytosis
- **C.** hyperglycemia
- **D.** marked elevations of serum amylase
- **E.** A, B, and C

180. Intraabdominal complications that might develop with this disease process include
- **A.** inflammatory pancreatic pseudocyst
- **B.** splenic vein thrombosis
- **C.** obstruction of the common bile duct
- **D.** acute gastrointestinal bleeding
- **E.** all of the above

Questions 181–183 (refer to Figure 2.32):

181. A patient with the barium swallow shown in Figure 2.32 is likely to experience all of the following except
- **A.** nocturnal pulmonary aspiration
- **B.** dumping syndrome
- **C.** dysphagia
- **D.** esophageal-oral regurgitation
- **E.** weight loss

182. The characteristic pathologic finding in this disorder is
- **A.** muscular thinning of the lower esophagus
- **B.** reduction or absence of ganglion cells in Auerbach's plexus
- **C.** intercellular muscular fibrosis
- **D.** Barrett's esophagus
- **E.** fatty infiltration

183. Optional therapeutic modalities for this disease include all of the following except
- **A.** nitrates
- **B.** lower esophageal pneumatic dilation
- **C.** esophageal myotomy
- **D.** calcium channel blockers
- **E.** metoclopramide

Questions 184–186 (refer to Figure 2.33):

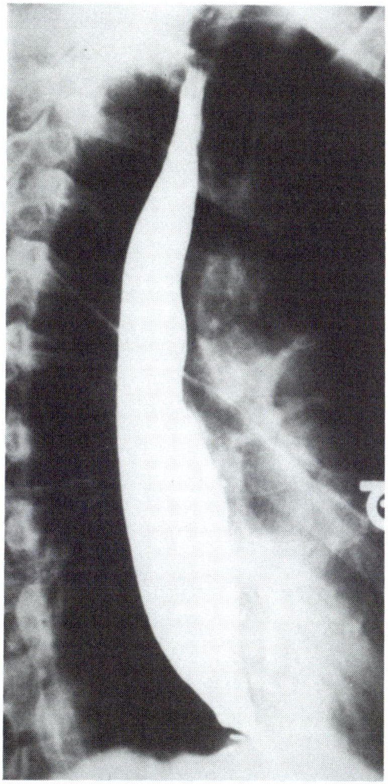

Figure 2.32

184. A 55-year-old man presents with a 1-month history of frontal headache that worsens considerably when he is supine. He has smoked two packs of cigarettes a day for 40 years and has a "smoker's cough." Physical examination reveals edema and dusky erythema of the face and neck and dilatation of the superficial veins of the upper extremities and chest. Chest radiograph is seen in Figure 2.33. This patient's clinical presentation is known as

B

A. Horner's syndrome
B. Pancoast's syndrome
C. superior vena cava syndrome
D. Eaton-Lambert syndrome
E. Trousseau's syndrome

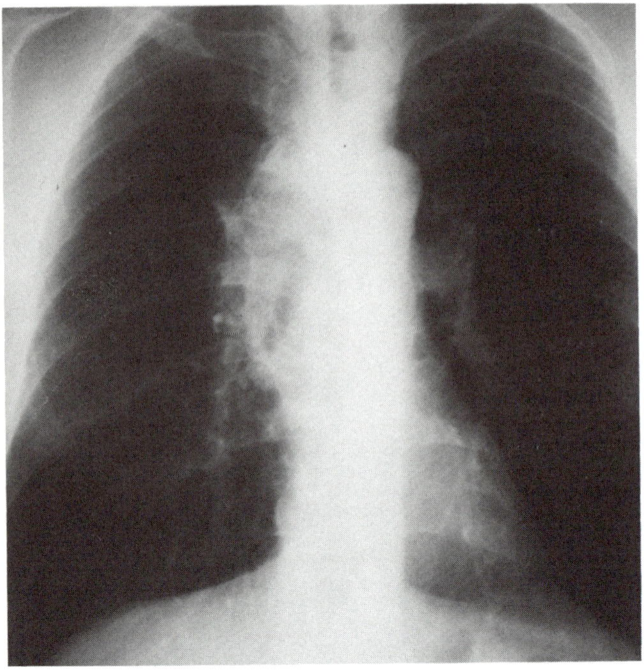

Figure 2.33

185. Bronchial biopsy during flexible fiberoptic bronchoscopy reveals small cell carcinoma of the lung. Paraneoplastic syndromes (ie, systemic effects of the tumor unrelated to metastases) associated with this particular cell type include all of the following except

A. SIADH
B. hypercalcemia from ectopic parathyroid hormone secretion
C. Cushing's syndrome from ectopic secretion of ACTH
D. gynecomastia
E. Eaton-Lambert (myasthenic) syndrome

186. In addition to a careful history, physical exam, and routine chemistries and complete blood count, appropriate pretreatment staging of the extent of disease in this patient with small cell carcinoma of the lung would include

- **A.** mediastinoscopy with biopsy, and, if negative for tumor, open thoracotomy
- **B.** flexible fiberoptic bronchoscopy, bone marrow biopsy, brain CT scan, and, if symptoms, physical exam, or laboratory findings are suggestive of disease involvement in these areas, radionuclide or CT scans of liver or bone
- **C.** radionuclide or CT scans of brain, liver, and bone even if routine evaluation suggests no metastases to these areas
- **D.** mediastinoscopy with biopsy and percutaneous or peritoneoscopy-directed liver biopsy
- **E.** none of the above

Questions 187–189 (refer to Figure 2.34):

187. A 36-year-old black woman presents with a 2-month history of intermittent fever, nonproductive cough, and vague anterior chest pain. The patient is currently afebrile, and the rest of her physical examination is normal. Her chest radiograph is seen in Figure 2.34. A differential diagnosis for this patient should include all of the following diseases except

- **A.** coccidioidomycosis
- **B.** tuberculosis
- **C.** sarcoidosis
- **D.** metastatic ovarian adenocarcinoma
- **E.** Hodgkin's disease

188. The most useful *initial* test to attempt to establish a diagnosis in this patient would be

- **A.** open lung biopsy
- **B.** mediastinoscopy and biopsy
- **C.** fiberoptic bronchoscopy with transbronchial biopsy
- **D.** serum angiotensin-converting enzyme (SACE) level
- **E.** Kveim-Siltzbach skin test

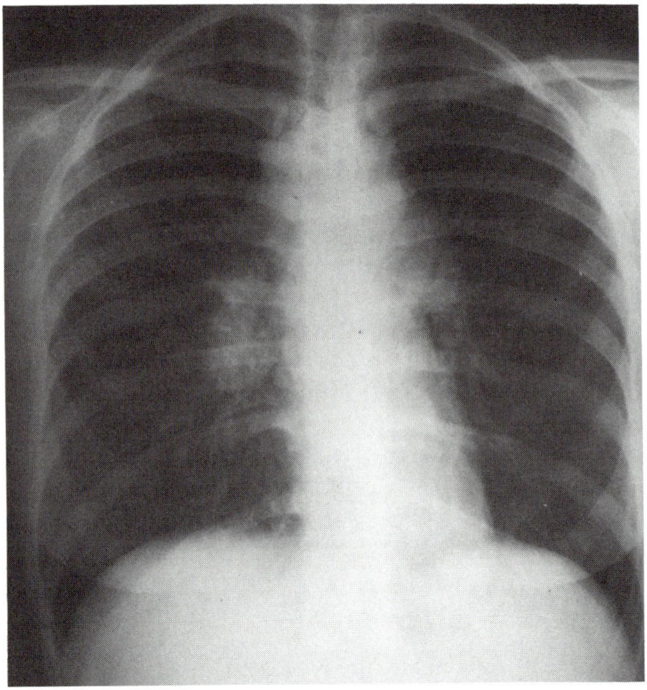

Figure 2.34

189. Tissue biopsy reveals noncaseating epithelioid granulomas for which fungal and mycobacterial cultures are negative. Usual indications for corticosteroid therapy for patients with this disorder include all of the following except

A. myocardial involvement (arrhythmias, heart failure)
B. ocular involvement (uveitis)
C. progressive worsening of pulmonary function
D. central nervous system abnormalities
E. arthritis and erythema nodosum

Questions 190–193 (refer to Figure 2.35):

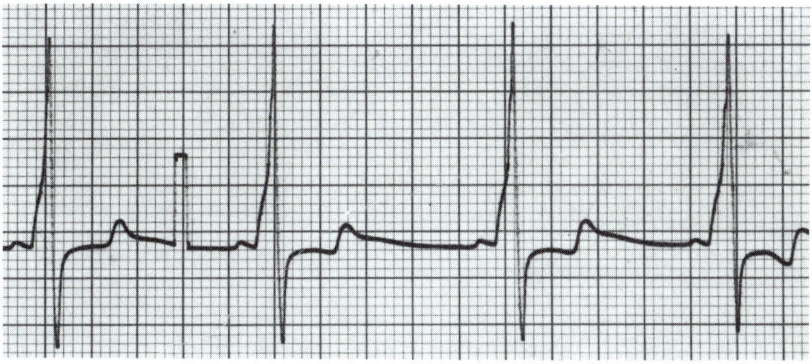

Figure 2.35

190. Patients with the ECG findings in Figure 2.35 may have which of the features listed below?

A. Paroxysmal supraventricular tachycardia (PSVT)
B. Atrial flutter and fibrillation with ventricular rates rapid enough to produce hypotension and/or sudden death
C. Ventricular tachycardia and sinus node dysfunction
D. No arrhythmias
E. All of the above

191. PSVT may be converted to sinus rhythm by all of the following maneuvers except

A. ice water facial immersion
B. hyperventilation
C. Valsalva
D. gagging
E. carotid sinus massage

192. Drugs that may be useful to prevent recurrence of PSVT include all of the following except

A. digoxin
B. verapamil
C. propranolol
D. quinidine
E. lidocaine

193. Which drug may be contraindicated as single therapy for prophylaxis of PSVT associated with ventricular preexcitation?

A. Quinidine
B. Digoxin
C. Amiodarone
D. Disopyramide
E. Procainamide

Questions 194–197 (refer to Figures 2.36 and 2.37):

Figure 2.36

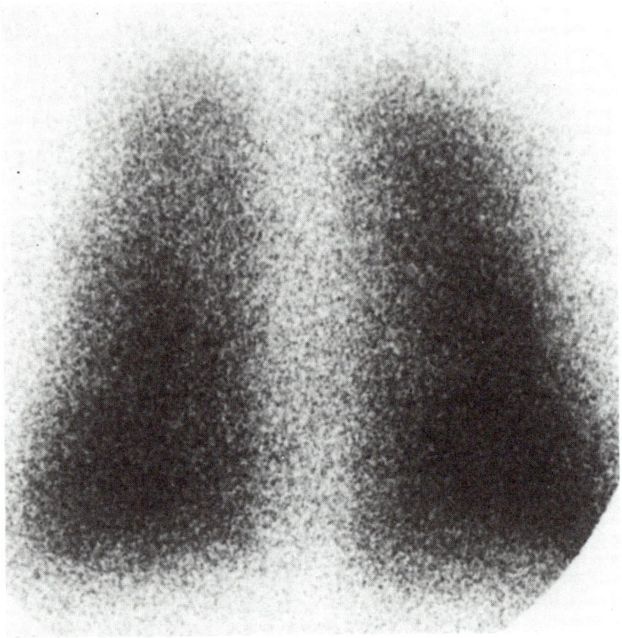

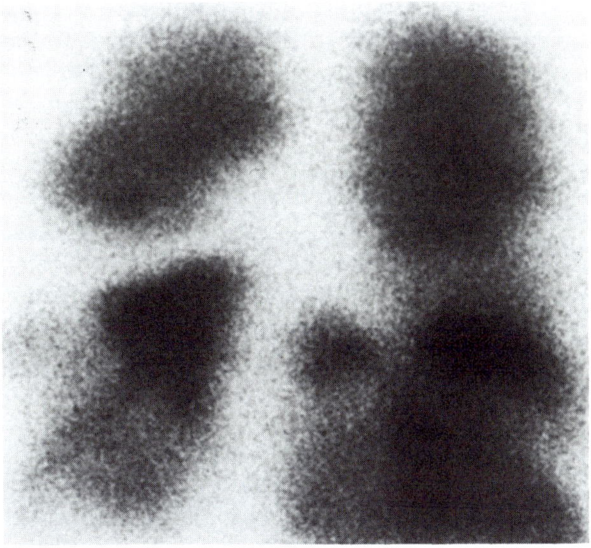

Figure 2.37

194. A 36-year-old woman is 9 weeks pregnant. She presents to the emergency room with severe dyspnea and anxiety of 4 hours duration. Physical exam reveals an anxious white woman with mild obesity, temperature = 36.5°C, respiratory rate = 28 breaths per minute, heart rate = 108 beats per minute, but is otherwise normal. The chest radiograph is normal. Room air (sea level) arterial blood gas shows $PaO_2 = 92$ torr, $PaCO_2 = 24$ torr, and pH = 7.53. An ECG shows sinus tachycardia, but is otherwise normal. This patient is not likely to have pulmonary embolism (PE) as the cause for her symptoms because

A. she has no clinical symptoms or signs of lower extremity deep vein thrombosis
B. she has a normal chest radiograph
C. she has a normal arterial PaO_2.
D. her ECG does not show evidence for right ventricular strain, for example, an $S_1Q_3T_3$ pattern with inverted T waves in leads V_1-V_3
E. none of the above

195. The ventilation (V) and perfusion (Q) scans in Figure 2.35 A and B, respectively, were obtained. The ventilation scan is normal and the perfusion scan shows multiple segmental defects; these findings are consistent with a high probability of PE. All of the following statements concerning V/Q scans are true except

- **A.** a normal perfusion scan rules out the diagnosis of PE
- **B.** a low probability V/Q scan pattern eliminates the need for pulmonary angiography to diagnose PE
- **C.** patients with a high probability V/Q scan pattern but at increased risk of hemorrhage with anticoagulant therapy should have pulmonary angiography to confirm the diagnosis of PE
- **D.** patients with severe obstructive lung disease most often have indeterminate V/Q scan patterns
- **E.** most patients with indeterminate V/Q scan patterns should undergo pulmonary angiography to confirm or deny the diagnosis of PE

196. All of the following statements concerning antithrombotic therapy for PE are true except

- **A.** initial therapy with thrombolytic agents instead of heparin is primarily reserved for patients with massive PE and hemodynamic instability
- **B.** because of the risk of hemorrhage, thrombolytic agents are absolutely contraindicated within 2 months of stroke or neurologic or ophthalmologic surgery, and are relatively contraindicated within 10 days of other surgery or internal organ biopsy
- **C.** patients receiving IV heparin must avoid concurrent therapy with antiplatelet agents such as aspirin and require monitoring of the platelet count
- **D.** warfarin therapy should be overlapped with heparin therapy for at least 4–5 days
- **E.** the optimal prothrombin time for long-term oral anticoagulation of PE is 1.5–2.0 times the control, that is, 18–24 seconds

197. Low dose subcutaneous heparin, 5000 U every 12 hours, significantly reduces the incidence of deep vein thrombosis and pulmonary embolism and should be used more often in all of the following clinical situations except

A. high-risk general surgery (patients over age 40 undergoing major thoracoabdominal procedures)
B. elective total hip replacement and surgical repair of traumatic hip fracture
C. genitourinary surgery for nonmalignant disorders
D. patients recovering from acute myocardial infarction
E. high-risk medical patients (congestive heart failure, thrombotic stroke, prolonged bed rest)

Questions 198–200 (refer to Figure 2.38):

198. A 25-year-old woman develops fever and substernal chest pain that is most intense when lying supine. The ST-segment abnormality shown in Figure 2.38 is present in the standard limb leads and in V_2-V_6. Seven days later, the T waves invert in the same leads. The most likely diagnosis is

A. Prinzmetal's angina
B. pulmonary embolus
C. Dressler's syndrome
D. acute pericarditis
E. mitral valve prolapse

199. This clinical entity may be found in all of the following except

A. infectious mononucleosis
B. uremia
C. tuberculosis
D. SLE
E. sprue

Figure 2.38

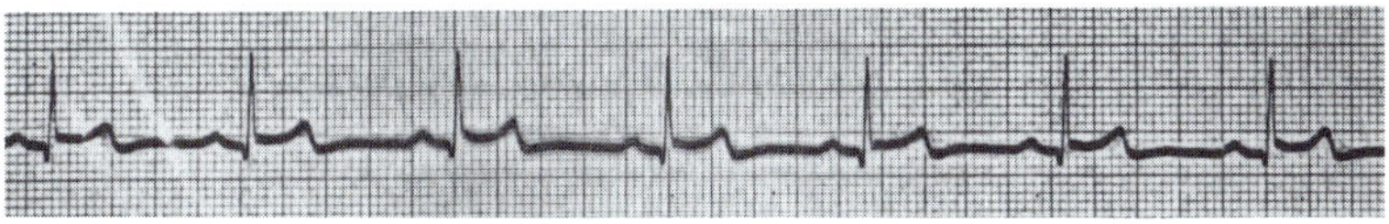

200. If the patient develops orthopnea with an elevated jugular venous pressure and faint heart sounds, appropriate therapy would be

A. furosemide 80 mg IV
B. placement of aortic counterpulsation balloon pump
C. IV nitroprusside
D. IV streptokinase
E. pericardiocentesis

Explanatory Answers

101. A. Hypochromic, microcytic blood cells can be seen in sideroblastic anemias, thalassemia, and anemia due to iron deficiency. Autoimmune hemolytic anemia is characterized by the presence of spherocytes in the peripheral blood, which appear as microcytic, hyperchromic cells. (Ref. 1, pp. 264, 265)

102. E. Decreased serum iron and an increased serum iron-binding capacity are characteristic of iron deficiency. Reduced plasma ferritin accurately reflects deficient iron stores. The platelet count can be increased or normal in iron deficiency anemia. (Ref. 1, pp. 1495–1497)

103. E. Iron deficiency results from decreased intake, increased requirements, decreased absorption, or blood loss. Pregnancy increases daily iron requirements three-fold. GI blood loss is the most important cause of iron deficiency in adult males, while menstrual blood loss is the most common cause in women of child-bearing age. Malabsorption, especially of the duodenum and jejunum, may result in iron deficiency. (Ref. 1, pp. 1493–1495)

104. C. Rouleaux formation and the presence of a nucleated red blood cell are shown in Figure 2.2. Rouleaux formation is secondary to excessive plasma globulins and may be seen in multiple myeloma. Bone marrow invasion (a myelophthisic process) can cause the early release of nucleated red blood cells into the peripheral blood. Alcoholic liver disease and vitamin B12 deficiency typically result in a macrocytosis, but not in rouleaux formation. (Ref. 2, pp. 900, 1028, 1029)

105. D. At the time of diagnosis, hypercalcemia is present in approximately one third of patients with multiple myeloma. Another one third develop elevated calcium levels during the course of the disease. Common symptoms include those listed, plus polyuria and polydipsia. Hyperglycemia, hyperuricemia, and hypokalemia are not commonly seen in multiple myeloma. (Ref. 8, p. 1773)

106. B. Normal saline and corticosteroids are often the first measures instituted for hypercalcemia. Antineoplastic therapy for myeloma should also be instituted. Insulin therapy and allopurinol are not useful in the treatment of hypercalcemia. (Ref. 8, p. 1773)

107. D. The abnormality depicted in Figure 2.3 is a *Plasmodium falciparum* gametocyte. Bartonellosis is an infection with *Bartonella bacilliformis*, a disease limited to certain valleys in the Andes mountains. Unlike these infections of red blood cells, Döhle bodies and toxic granulations are abnormalities of neutrophils found in infections and other toxic states. (Ref. 1, pp. 620, 778, 779)

108. C. Treatment for all types of acute malaria, except drug-resistant falciparum, can be achieved with chloroquine. Due to the emergence of drug-resistant falciparum in Southeast Asia and South America, acute infections of falciparum require the use of combination therapy, including quinine, pyrimethamine, and use of the sulfonamides or sulfones. High-dose corticosteroids and broad spectrum antibiotics have not been found to be of benefit in the treatment of acute malaria. (Ref. 1, pp. 782, 783)

109. A. Chloroquine is effective in preventing the primary episodes of *P. vivax* and *P. ovale.* In areas endemic for chloroquine-resistant *P. falciparum*, weekly Fansidar (pyrimethamine, 25 mg and sulfadoxine, 500 mg) should be used concurrently. The vector, the Anopheles mosquito, should be avoided by netting, repellents, and proper clothing. The tsetse fly is important in the transmission of African trypanosomiasis, not malaria. (Ref. 2, pp. 1860–1862)

110. A. The peripheral blood smear in disseminated intravascular coagulation (DIC) is characterized by the presence of schistocytes, helmet cells, and decreased platelets. Multiple conditions, including malignancies, vascular malformations and thrombosis, infections, and retained fetus and amniotic fluid, are associated with DIC. Prosthetic valve hemolysis is not associated with thrombocytopenia. (Ref. 1, pp. 1511, Plate A5-7)

111. B. Impaired coagulation, including prolonged prothrombin time, decreased plasma fibrinogen, and thrombocytopenia, are seen in DIC and in chronic liver disease. Anemia, multifactorial in nature, may be seen in patients with alcoholic liver disease. Surreptitious heparin use is typically manifested by an elevated partial thromboplastin time, without other abnormalities of hemostasis. An isolated elevation of the prothrombin time is found in patients with a vitamin K deficiency. (Ref. 1, pp. 1478–1483)

112. A. Acute promyelocytic leukemia is associated with DIC, especially during induction of chemotherapy. Heparin appears to be superior to warfarin in treating DIC, and is often used prophylactically during induction therapy of acute promyelocytic leukemia. Therapy for underlying acidosis or infection should always be instituted. DIC associated with malignancy usually requires treatment of the malignancy. Steroids are generally not utilized for acute promyelocytic leukemia and secondary DIC. (Ref. 2, pp. 1078, 1079, 1098)

113. B. Homosexual or bisexual men, IV drug abusers, Haitians, patients with hemophilia A, and sexual partners of AIDS patients are at high risk to develop AIDS. Household contacts of AIDS patients and medical personnel caring for AIDS patients are at very low risk of contracting AIDS, provided they avoid contact with the patient's blood and other body secretions. (Ref. 1, pp. 1392, 1393)

114. C. The presence of interstitial infiltrates in a patient with AIDS is most likely due to *P. carinii*. The subacute course is also consistent with cytomegalovirus or other viral pneumonias. The chest x-ray in pneumococcal pneumonia is characterized by focal alveolar infiltrates rather then diffuse interstitial infiltrates. *Cryptosporidium* may cause severe diarrhea in AIDS patients, but does not affect the lung. (Ref. 1, pp. 797, 798)

115. C. Pentamidine and trimethoprim-sulfamethoxazole have been shown to be effective in the treatment of *P. carinii*, which is seen in Figure 2.5. *P. carinii* organisms are not sensitive to either erythromycin or acyclovir. (Ref. 6, 7: x: 16, 17)

116. C. The patient's history is classic for disseminated gonococcal disease. Blood cultures and direct fluorescent antibody staining of skin lesion scrapings can establish the diagnosis in over 50% of cases during the early stage of dissemination. Joint fluid is usually sterile during the initial stage of disseminated gonococcemia. The diagnosis is more readily established by immunofluorescent staining of skin lesions rather than by culture of the scrapings. (Ref. 1, p. 579)

117. A. During the later stages of disseminated gonococcemia, the synovial culture is positive in at least 50% of cases. Pharyngeal and rectal cultures will establish the diagnosis in some additional cases. Blood cultures are rarely positive in the later stage. (Ref. 1, pp. 579, 580)

118. A. *Neisseria* strains grow on the selective Thayer-Martin medium, and both *N. meningitidis* and *N. gonorrhoeae* yield positive oxidase reactions. *N. gonorrhoeae* metabolizes glucose but not maltose. (Ref. 2, p. 1611)

119. B. These two regimens are effective in disseminated gonococcemia. One-time-only procaine penicillin and 7 days of oral tetracycline are effective in uncomplicated anogenital infections in heterosexuals, but not in disseminated gonococcemia. (Ref. 1, p. 581)

120. E. The endocervix and urethra, at a rate of almost 80% to 90%, are the most commonly involved sites of infection. Approximately one half of women with gonorrhea are minimally symptomatic or asymptomatic. Presenting symptoms include vaginal discharge, hemorrhage, or may mimic cystitis caused by Gram-negative bacilli. The major complication of PID is infertility, estimated to be 15% after one episode, and about 50% after three episodes. (Ref. 2, pp. 1707, 1708)

121. C. The peripheral blood smear is significant for macrocytic oval red blood cells (macroovalocytes) and a polymorphonuclear leukocyte with a hypersegmented nucleus. These changes are seen in the megaloblastic anemias secondary to vitamin B12 and folate deficiencies. Chronic blood loss and iron deficiency are characterized by microcytic, hypochromic red cell morphology. Sickle cell anemia is manifest by both normocytic and sickled cells on examination of the peripheral blood. (Ref. 1, Plate A5-6, Plate A5-18; Ref. 2, pp. 881, 882, 900–907, 936–942)

122. A. Because the patient has a macrocytic anemia, evaluation would include both vitamin B12 and folate levels. Stool guaiacs would be an essential element in the evaluation of any anemia.

Hemoglobin electrophoresis would not be indicated in this patient with a macrocytic anemia. (Ref. 1, pp. 263, 1502, 1503)

123. A. A deficiency of intrinsic factor, or diseases involving the terminal ileum (regional enteritis), the site of vitamin B12 absorption, can result in vitamin B12 deficiency. The Schilling test helps to delineate the etiology of vitamin B12 deficiency. (Ref. 1, pp. 1500–1502)

124. D. The myeloblast shown contains an Auer rod, seen only in myeloblasts of acute granulocytic leukemia. Myeloblasts seen in chronic granulocytic leukemia in blast crisis lack Auer rods. The malignant cells found in chronic lymphocytic leukemia resemble mature lymphocytes. Lymphoblasts in acute lymphoblastic leukemia have a high nuclear cytoplasmic ratio and lack Auer rods. (Ref. 1, pp. 1543, 1544, Plates A5-22–A5-24)

125. B. Myeloblasts stain positively with Sudan B black stain and myeloperoxidase. The Philadelphia chromosome (a reciprocal translocation of a portion of the long arm of chromosome 22, usually to chromosome 9) is found in over 90% of patients with chronic granulocytic leukemia. Elevated terminal deoxynucleotidyl transferase is found in T and null-cell types of acute lymphoblastic leukemia. (Ref. 1, p. 1543; Ref. 2, pp. 989, 1002, 1003)

126. B. An age greater than 70 years, chromosomal abnormalities (−5, −7, t(9;22)), a history of preleukemia, and a monoblastic component are all associated with a poorer prognosis. Patients with translocations t(8;21) + t(15;17) or promyelocytic leukemia generally exhibit increased survival. (Ref. 1, pp. 1546, 1547)

127. E. The clinical history and loss of haustra with narrowing of the left colon suggest ulcerative colitis. GI complications include all of the answers listed in addition to colonic perforation, colonic stricture, rectal prolapse, and massive colonic hemorrhage. (Ref. 15, pp. 1148–1155)

128. C. Some authorities have advocated prophylactic colectomy to prevent colon cancer in patients with universal colitis of more than 10-years duration. An alternative option is careful surveillance colonoscopy to obtain multiple sequential biopsies assessing for mucosal dysplasia. Anticholinergic drugs and opiates are generally not effective in controlling diarrhea in the setting of severe colitis and actually may contribute to the development of toxic megacolon. Infectious colitis may mimic ulcerative colitis. (Ref. 15, pp. 1136, 1137, 1144, 1154)

129. A. Articular manifestations are present in approximately 25% of patients with IBD over the course of their disease. A monoarticular or polyarticular form commonly involves knees, ankles, and wrists and parallels the activity of the bowel disease. The central arthritis (ankylosing spondylitis) is not related to the course of the underlying bowel diseases. (Ref. 1, p. 1286)

130. D. The clinical course of pyoderma gangrenosum typically parallels the activity of colitis. Corticosteroids, sulfasalazine, and dapsone may be effective medical treatment, but refractory severe pyoderma gangrenosum is an indication for colectomy. Grafting and vigorous debridement should be avoided as these may aggravate the disease. No benefit has been reported with penicillin or with the antifungal agent ketoconazole. (Ref. 5, pp. 478–481)

131. D. Serial chest radiographs are not cost-effective in the follow-up of patients with positive PPDs. As the patient under discussion is likely to receive chronic, high dose steroid therapy, treatment with isoniazid for 1 year is indicated. Rifampin is indicated for 1 year for a new PPD converter if the patient has been exposed to a source case infected with tubercle bacilli documented to be resistant to isoniazid. Once a patient demonstrates a positive reaction to PPD, repeat PPD testing is contraindicated as this may result in severe local tissue necrosis. (Ref. 1, pp. 631, 632)

132. B. There is a 3%–5% incidence of hepatitis in patients taking isoniazid and rifampin. Induction of P-450 cytochrome system by drugs such as alcohol or barbiturates predispose to isoniazid hepatitis. The hepatitis usually resolves with prompt discontinuation of the drug. A reversible peripheral neuropathy, associated with isoniazid use, can be prevented or treated with pyridoxine. Influenza-like syndrome and thrombocytopenia are seen with rifampin, not isoniazid. (Ref. 1, pp. 631, 632)

133. A. Atrial flutter is usually associated with a variety of organic heart diseases, but may also be seen with pericardial disease and a variety of metabolic disorders. Quinidine toxicity is most frequently manifested as bradyarrhythmias, conduction disturbances, and ventricular arrhythmias. (Ref. 9, pp. 629, 671, 672)

134. C. In contrast to atrial fibrillation, the atria contract during atrial flutter, which may account for the lesser incidence of systemic emboli associated with atrial flutter. Because they slow the rate of atrial contraction and enhance AV-node conduction, type I antiarrhythmics (quinidine, disopyramide, and procainamide) may increase the ventricular response rate in patients with atrial flutter, converting 2:1 atrioventricular conduction to 1:1 conduction; this may be prevented by coadministration of digoxin, propranolol, or verapamil. Carotid sinus massage rarely converts atrial flutter to sinus rhythm. DC cardioversion with low energies (≤50 joules) will frequently convert atrial flutter to sinus rhythm. (Ref. 9, pp. 671, 672)

135. A. Electrocardioversion may produce ventricular fibrillation, asystole, and a variety of other arrhythmias. Embolic episodes occur in 1%–3% of patients converted to sinus rhythm; patients with a history of emboli, mitral stenosis, a prosthetic mitral valve, or an enlarged heart are at relatively high risk for emboli. Elevations of myocardial enzymes after cardioversion are uncommon and generally occur after multiple high-energy countershocks. Cardioversion does not result in pericarditis. (Ref. 9, pp. 643, 644)

136. B. Tuberculous and fungal meningitis typically have mild to moderate elevation of CSF protein, decreased CSF glucose, and an elevated leukocyte count; in contrast to bacterial meningitis, the leukocytes in the CSF are predominantly lymphocytes. In subarachnoid hemorrhage, the CSF is usually extremely bloody. (Ref. 1, pp. 737, 738, 1982)

137. D. This figure shows a positive india ink preparation for *Cryptococcus neoformans*. CT scans of the brain, or technetium brain scans, only occasionally reveal focal lesions and would require serologic or culture confirmation of this diagnosis. Blood cultures are positive in 10% of patients. Virtually all patients with cryptococcal meningoencephalitis will have detectable capsular antigen in CSF or serum. (Ref. 1, pp. 737, 738)

138. A. Cryptococcal meningoencephalitis requires treatment with IV amphotericin B, either alone or in combination with oral flucytosine. Amphotericin routinely results in renal insufficiency and hypokalemia. Flucytosine is associated with neutropenia, thrombocytopenia, and colitis. Treatment for at least 6 weeks, with four consecutive sterile weekly cultures, results in cure 50%–70% of the time. Peripheral neuropathy is seen with isoniazid therapy. (Ref. 1, pp. 737, 738)

139. E. The patient in Figure 2.13 has a purpuric rash due to meningococcemia. Altered mental status, fever, and a petechial or purpuric rash may be seen in all of the listed conditions. (Ref. 1, pp. 575, 576)

140. A. Counterimmunoelectrophoresis or latex agglutination of spinal fluid may be useful in rapidly establishing the diagnosis of meningococcal meningitis. The organism may be recovered from cultures of blood, spinal fluid, or petechial scrapings. The presence of meningococcus in the nasopharynx does not, by itself, establish the diagnosis of meningococcal infection. (Ref. 1, pp. 575, 576)

141. A. Intimate contacts of patients with meningococcal disease should receive prophylaxis with rifampin or minocycline in the doses given. Sulfonamides may be used for organisms known to be sensitive to sulfonamides. Penicillin VK has not been shown to provide effective prophylaxis for meningococcal disease. (Ref. 1, p. 576)

142. D. Figure 2.14 demonstrates bony enlargement and spur formation along the distal interphalangeal joints (Heberden's nodes) and proximal interphalangeal joints (Bouchard's nodes) of the fingers characteristic of osteoarthritis. The ESR is normal in most patients. (Ref. 12, pp. 42, 44, 106, 107)

143. B. Therapy for osteoarthritis includes aspirin or nonsteroidal antiinflammatory agents to relieve pain and decrease inflammation. Corticosteroids are usually ineffective in improving symptoms from osteoarthritis. Isometric exercises are more likely to maintain muscle function and strength without aggravating joint symptoms than are isotonic exercises against resistance. (Ref. 12, p. 107)

144. E. Clubbing may be a finding in each of these disorders. (Ref. 12, p. 168)

145. A. Hypertrophic osteoarthropathy may include all of the manifestations listed in 1 to 3. While this disorder may sometimes be mistaken for rheumatoid arthritis, it is not associated with rheumatoid nodule formation. (Ref. 12, p. 168)

146. E. The radiograph in Figure 2.16 demonstrates calcification of the articular cartilage of the knee joint consistent with calcium pyrophosphate deposition disease (chondrocalcinosis). Patients with this disorder may present with any of the listed clinical patterns. (Ref. 12, pp. 128–130)

147. D. These are calcium pyrophosphate dihydrate crystals and are frequently found in the joint fluid of patients with calcium pyrophosphate deposition disease. A positive synovial bacterial culture and glucose concentration less than 50% of a simultaneously measured serum glucose level are frequent findings in acute bacterial arthritis. The crystals in answer 2 are uric acid crystals found in gouty arthritis. (Ref. 1, pp. 1459, 1463)

148. E. Figure 2.17 demonstrates swelling and erythema of the metatarsophalangeal joint of the great toe. Acute monoarticular arthritis of this joint is the most common initial presentation of gout, when it is called podagra. However, the other diagnoses listed, and also trauma, acute sarcoidosis, and psoriatic arthritis, may present with a similar acute monoarticular arthritis ("pseudopodagra"). (Ref. 2, p. 1168)

149. D. Colchicine or nonsteroidal antiinflammatory drugs will relieve acute gouty arthritis in a majority of patients. Modalities that lower serum urate—probenecid, allopurinol, and low purine diet—are of no value in the treatment of the acute attack and may even precipitate acute gouty arthritis. (Ref. 2, pp. 1168, 1169)

150. D. Only the presence of intraleukocytic sodium urate crystals in aspirated joint fluid establishes a diagnosis of gout. While suggestive, the individual findings of hyperuricemia, podagra, or response to colchicine therapy are not pathognomonic of gout. (Ref. 1, p. 1626)

151. C. Variegation of color and irregular borders are characteristic of malignant melanoma. Suspicious colors include shades of red, white, or blue, sometimes mixed with black or brown. Nodularity or ulceration characteristically develop in the course of a progressive, malignant melanoma. (Ref. 1, p. 1595)

152. C. It is thought that persons who tan poorly or who have a history of blistering burns in childhood are at increased risk of developing malignant melanoma. There is an inverse relationship between latitude and melanoma incidence; incidence rates are twice as great in the southwestern United States as in the northeast. No link has been established between chronic suntanning and melanoma. Patients with large, congenital melanocytic nevi are at risk to develop melanoma in the lesion. (Ref. 1, p. 1596)

153. A. The spider angioma shown in Figure 2.19 is frequently found in association with cirrhosis, which may be clinically manifested by ascites, jaundice, anorexia, splenomegaly, gynecomastia, testicular atrophy, amenorrhea, clubbing, and loss of body hair (rather than hirsutism). (Ref. 1, p. 1342)

154. C. Hepatitis B and non-A, non-B hepatitis may result in cirrhosis, whereas CMV and hepatitis A infections may cause hepatitis but do not progress to cirrhosis. (Ref. 1, pp. 698, 699, 1332, 1343)

155. B. PSE may be precipitated by GI bleeding, increased dietary protein, hypokalemic alkalosis, infections, and progressive deterioration of liver function. A diet high in carbohydrates and low in protein is useful in the treatment of PSE. Vitamin K administration may occasionally improve the coagulopathy in patients with liver disease, but would not affect PSE. (Ref. 1, pp. 1349–1351)

156. A. Oral neomycin and lactulose therapy decrease ammonia production and absorption in the bowel. Protein restriction and control of GI bleeding will also decrease production of ammonia and other nitrogenous substances in the colon. Correction of electrolyte abnormalities is important and all CNS depressants should be avoided because these agents may exacerbate PSE. (Ref. 1, pp. 1350, 1351)

157. C. *Giardia lamblia* is a commonly identified pear-shaped protozoan with two distinctive nuclei; humans, dogs, beavers, and other mammals are natural hosts. Infection is acquired by ingestion of cysts excreted in stool or by direct person-to-person fecal contamination. Male homosexuals have a high rate of intestinal parasitosis, including *G. lamblia*. Typhoid fever is caused by the bacterium *Salmonella typhi*. (Ref. 15, pp. 940, 986, 987)

158. B. Giardiasis frequently accompanies IgA and IgM immunoglobulin deficiencies. The pathogenesis of diarrhea and steatorrhea is unknown. Fecal leukocytes are frequently found in bacterial diarrhea but not in giardiasis. In contrast to many other parasitic diseases, eosinophilia is not a feature of giardiasis. (Ref. 15, pp. 986, 987)

159. C. Figure 2.21 shows a red blood cell (RBC) cast indicative of glomerular injury; these casts typically have a reddish hue when observed by light microscopy. The patient has acute glomerulonephritis (GLN): gross hematuria with proteinuria, hypertension, edema, and azotemia. Primary renal diseases that present as acute GLN include those listed in answer 2. Bacterial endocarditis, visceral abscesses, other nonbacterial infections, and systemic diseases such as systemic lupus erythematosus, may also present as acute GLN. Membranous nephropathy and MCNS present as nephrotic syndrome (heavy proteinuria [$>$3.5 g/day], hypoalbuminemia, edema, and hyperlipidemia) rather than acute GLN; the onset is insidious rather than acute and RBC casts and gross hematuria are infrequent. Obstructive uropathy from renal calculi would not result in RBC casts. (Ref. 2, pp. 582–592)

160. E. ASO titers are increased in 70% and the streptozyme test is positive in 95% of patients with poststreptococcal GLN. Serum levels of C_3 and/or C_4 are reduced with certain types of GLN and may be helpful diagnostically. Anti-GBM antibodies are present in patients with Goodpasture's syndrome and anti-GBM antibody-mediated renal disease. Blood cultures assist in the diagnosis of bacterial endocarditis as a cause of acute GLN. (Ref. 2, pp. 584, 587, 589, 590)

161. E. The radiograph in Figure 2.22 reveals ankylosing spondylitis involving the lumbosacral spine and pelvis (there is also residual dye from a myelogram). There are syndesmophytes (ossification of the annulus fibrosus and paravertebral ligaments) involving both lateral surfaces of the intervertebral disks that bridge adjacent vertebrae. Both sacroiliac joints are narrowed and sclerosed. Ankylosing spondylitis results in anterior flexion of the thoracolumbar spine and is accompanied by episodes of acute anterior uveitis in 20%–30% of patients and by peripheral arthritis of the hips and shoulders in 25% of patients. Ninety percent of patients with ankylosing spondylitis have the HLA-B27 antigen. (Ref. 1, pp. 1434–1436)

162. C. Nonsteroidal antiinflammatory agents are useful to alleviate pain and stiffness and thereby facilitate maintenance of erect posture through exercise and physical therapy. Gold therapy is not useful, and corticosteroid therapy is usually indicated only for severe anterior uveitis. (Ref. 1, p. 1436)

163. E. The chest radiograph in Figure 2.23 shows a large lung abscess in the right midlung field; a lateral film (not shown) located the lesion to the superior segment of the right lower lobe. The most common etiology of lung abscess is anaerobic infection, for which aspiration and periodontal sepsis (eg, gingivitis, pyorrhea) are the most important predisposing factors. Aspiration may occur with altered consciousness due to alcoholism, drug addiction or overdose, or general anesthesia. Dysphagia from esophageal or neurologic disease may also result in aspiration. Periodontal sepsis increases the quantity of relatively virulent anaerobic bacteria in the mouth. (Ref. 2, pp. 435, 436)

164. A. Lung abscess may result from primary anaerobic infection, certain aerobic bacteria (especially *Staphylococcus aureus, Klebsiella pneumoniae*, and *Streptococcus pyogenes*), tuberculous or fungal infection, amebiasis, or an obstructing bronchogenic carcinoma. Isolated pneumococcal pneumonia in the absence of other organisms is at best a rare cause of lung abscess. (Ref. 2, pp. 435, 436)

165. A. The bacterial organisms listed are anaerobes commonly found in patients with anaerobic lung abscess. The most commonly used antibiotic is penicillin G in an IV dose of 10–20 million U/day. Because penicillin-resistant anaerobes, including

Bacteroides melaninogenicus, are found in 25% of anaerobic lung abscesses, some clinicians prefer clindamycin or penicillin G combined with metronidazole as the treatment of choice. Aminoglycosides such as gentamicin have very little activity against anaerobes and should not be used to treat anaerobic lung abscess. (Ref. 2, pp. 437, 438)

166. D. The ECG reveals ST-segment elevation in V1-V6 with Q waves in V2-V6 consistent with an acute anterolateral myocardial infarction. Myocardial infarction may present in the elderly as new or increased congestive heart failure, stroke, syncope, weakness, confusion, and/or hypotension in the absence of chest pain. Pulmonary embolus and acute myocarditis may produce nonspecific ST-segment depression and/or T-wave inversion, but not ST-segment elevation and Q waves. Pericarditis may result in striking ST-segment elevation but would not produce the Q waves seen in this ECG. The ECG in patients with dissection of the descending aorta generally shows no acute changes; dissection of the ascending aorta may cause acute myocardial infarction. (Ref. 1, pp. 980, 982, 983, 1003, 1009, 1039)

167. E. Pulmonary embolus may be accompanied by ST-segment depression and/or T-wave inversion, but not by ST-segment elevation. Transient ST-segment elevation secondary to myocardial ischemia occurs with myocardial infarction and coronary artery spasm. Pericarditis may be associated with epicardial myocarditis, which may produce diffuse ST-segment elevation. Persistent ST-segment elevation may indicate the presence of a ventricular aneurysm. (Ref. 11, pp. 212, 986, 1108)

168. E. Myocardial infarction does not predispose to endocarditis but may be complicated by the other clinical features listed, as well as by ventricular aneurysm formation, cardiac rupture, and septal perforation. (Ref. 9, pp. 1264, 1265, 1283–1287)

169. D. The patient is in cardiogenic shock, and dopamine should be employed for immediately life-threatening hypotension with the goal of maintaining a systolic pressure between 80 and 100 mmHg. Hemodynamic monitoring would subsequently be essential to maintain the pulmonary capillary wedge pressure in a desirable range (15–18 mmHg) for optimal left ventricular function. IV saline may precipitate or exacerbate congestive heart failure in this patient. Digitalis and furosemide are not effective therapy for cardiogenic shock. Pericardiocentesis is indicated only if cardiac tamponade from pericardial effusion is suspected. (Ref. 14, pp. 111–119)

170. D. The rhythm strip demonstrates ventricular tachycardia. Immediate DC cardioversion should be attempted in an unconscious monitored patient with ventricular tachycardia. An initial precordial thump may be given while charging the defibrillator. A second countershock with another 200 joules should be attempted if the first countershock is unsuccessful. Lidocaine or bretylium is administered after cardioversion, whether successful or unsuccessful. The value of sodium bicarbonate is questionable during the cardiac arrest, and it is not recommended for routine cardiac arrest sequences. (Ref. 20, pp. 2946, 2947)

171. D. The ECG shows atrial fibrillation and the chest radiograph demonstrates cardiomegaly and massive left atrial enlargement (manifest by a double density sign, elevation of the left main-stem bronchus, and a protuberant left heart border). This degree of left atrial enlargement is highly suggestive of mitral valve disease. Coronary artery disease, hyperthyroidism, sick sinus syndrome, and pulmonary embolus may all cause atrial fibrillation, but would not generally be associated with such prominent left atrial enlargement. (Ref. 9, pp. 673, 1030)

172. A. Appropriate initial therapy is to slow the ventricular rate to 60–80 beats/min; digoxin is preferable to propranolol as it will not exacerbate underlying heart failure and may be administered once daily. Atrial fibrillation associated with mitral valve disease is accompanied by a significantly increased risk of cerebral embolism, and unless contraindicated, this patient should be anticoagulated. DC cardioversion should not be attempted until the patient has been anticoagulated for 2–4 weeks, and may not be successful long term with this degree of left atrial enlargement. Lidocaine and bretylium are useful for ventricular but not atrial arrhythmias. (Ref. 9, pp. 627, 635, 673, 674)

173. C. The ECG shows a regular rhythm with inverted P waves following the QRS complex consistent with a nonparoxysmal junctional rhythm, that is, a form of third degree heart block. Digoxin toxicity frequently causes this rhythm and may have been precipitated here by the doubling of the serum digoxin level, which usually follows initiation of maintenance quinidine therapy. The other answers do not cause third degree heart block. Hypocalcemia prolongs the ST segment and QT interval, while hypercalcemia shortens them. Hypokalemia prolongs the QT interval, flattens the T wave, and may depress the ST segment. Hypomagnesemia cannot be recognized on the ECG. (Ref. 9, pp. 216–218, 500)

174. C. Cholestyramine and neomycin decrease digoxin absorption and serum digoxin levels, thereby diminishing the risk of digoxin toxicity; nifedipine has no effect on serum digoxin level. Verapamil and amiodarone increase serum digoxin levels 70%–100% and may precipitate digoxin toxicity. Hypokalemia, hypomagnesemia, hypercalcemia, hypoxemia, hypercapnia, and increasing severity of heart disease all predispose the myocardium to the toxic effects of digoxin. (Ref. 9, pp. 500–503)

175. A. Quinidine and procainamide are not first-line agents for treating arrhythmias due to digitalis intoxication, as they may further depress cardiac conduction and contractility; quinidine also increases serum digoxin concentration. Potassium is useful to treat tachyarrhythmias, especially in hypokalemic patients, but should be avoided or used with great caution in patients with AV-nodal block, which may be worsened by potassium therapy. Lidocaine and phenytoin do not depress cardiac conduction and are useful in the treatment of tachyarrhythmias caused by digitalis excess. Atropine or electrical pacing may be required for symptomatic bradyarrhythmias. Digoxin-specific antibodies are helpful for patients with severe digitalis intoxication. (Ref. 9, pp. 506, 507)

176. B. The gross pathologic specimen reveals multiple polypoid lesions that histologically proved to be adenomas. Familial polyposis coli is an inherited autosomal dominant trait characterized by the presence of hundreds, or even thousands, of adenomatous polyps in the colon. Peutz-Jeghers syndrome, juvenile polyposis, and Cowden's syndrome are familial hamartomatous, rather than adenomatous, polyposis syndromes. The polypoid lesions in pneumatosis cystoides intestinalis are actually air-filled cysts within the submucosa of the colon, rather than true polyps. (Ref. 15, pp. 1207–1216)

177. D. Colon cancer typically occurs 10–15 years after the onset of the polyposis in familial polyposis coli. Diligent surveillance of relatives is mandatory for colon cancer prevention. Subtotal colectomy with ileorectal anastomosis may be acceptable therapy in patients without rectal polyps who agree to careful follow-up. Familial polyposis coli is not associated with ulcerative colitis or liver disease. While these patients may experience bowel obstruction from intussusception associated with large polyps, or hematochezia from polyp bleeding, these complications by themselves do not mandate total proctocolectomy. (Ref. 15, pp. 1210–1212)

178. E. The abdominal radiograph in Figure 2.31 reveals diffuse pancreatic calcification. This occurs in the setting of chronic pancreatitis, which in the United States is most often secondary to alcohol abuse. Other causes of chronic pancreatitis, protein malnutrition, hyperparathyroidism, and islet-cell tumors, are all causes of pancreatic calcification. (Ref. 1, p. 1378)

179. E. Chronic pancreatitis that is complicated by significant loss of exocrine and endocrine function may consequently give rise to diabetes mellitus and fat malabsorption, as well as vitamin B12 malabsorption. Macrocytosis may appear secondary to B12 deficiency and/or concurrent ethanol-induced liver disease or folate deficiency. Serum amylase levels are usually not elevated. (Ref. 15, pp. 1490–1492)

180. E. Pancreatic pseudocysts, splenic vein thrombosis, and obstruction of the pancreatic portion of the common bile duct are all potential complications of chronic pancreatitis. Acute gastrointestinal bleeding in these patients may result from hemorrhage of a pancreatic pseudocyst into the stomach, duodenum, or pancreatic duct, or from gastric varices that may complicate splenic vein thrombosis. (Ref. 15, pp. 1498–1503)

181. B. The barium swallow is indicative of achalasia, typically associated with the distal esophageal narrowing that represents a nonrelaxing lower esophageal sphincter and esophageal dilatation proximal to the narrowing. Usual symptoms include regurgitation, dysphagia, and chest pain associated with progressive weight loss. Dumping syndrome (postprandial abdominal cramps, vomiting, diarrhea, dizziness, and weakness) is a complication of surgery for peptic ulcer, not of achalasia. (Ref. 15, pp. 169, 760–763)

182. B. In most cases of achalasia, the ganglion cells are markedly reduced in number. This supports the hypothesis that denervation of the inhibitory nerves in the lower esophageal sphincter is the cause of the elevated lower esophageal sphincter pressure. The lower esophagus typically reveals muscular thickening without fibrosis or fatty infiltration. Barrett's esophagus is characterized by columnarization of the normally squamous esophageal epithelium, and is associated with gastroesophageal reflux rather than achalasia. (Ref. 15, p. 431)

183. E. Nitrates and calcium channel blockers have been reported to decrease lower esophageal sphincter (LES) pressure. Hydrostatic or pneumatic dilatation of the LES and incision of the circular muscle fibers down to the mucosa may also be efficacious. Metoclopramide is a dopamine antagonist that is utilized in gastroesophageal reflux patients to elevate the lower esophageal sphincter pressure, which would be undesirable in achalasia. (Ref. 15, pp. 437–439, 468)

184. C. The chest radiograph in Figure 2.33 shows a mass lesion in the upper portion of the right hilum and the right paratracheal region of the mediastinum. The mass has compressed the superior vena cava and increased the pressure in this vein and its tributaries in the head, chest, and upper extremities resulting in edema, cyanosis, and dilatation of superficial veins in these regions. Bronchogenic carcinoma (especially small cell carcinoma, which was the diagnosis in this case), lymphomas, and a variety of other benign disorders may all produce the superior vena cava syndrome. Pancoast tumors are bronchogenic carcinomas arising in the subpleural region of the superior sulcus; they may give rise to Horner's syndrome (ptosis, miosis, and decreased facial sweating on the affected side) due to pressure on the stellate ganglion. The Eaton-Lambert (myasthenic) syndrome may be seen with small cell lung cancer. Trousseau's syndrome of migratory venous thrombophlebitis may also be seen with bronchogenic carcinoma. (Ref. 1, p. 1117; Ref. 16, pp. 812, 813)

185. B. Hypercalcemia from ectopic parathyroid hormone secretion is associated with epidermoid (squamous cell) carcinoma of the lung rather than small cell carcinoma. The other paraneoplastic syndromes listed are seen with small cell carcinoma. (Ref. 1, p. 1117)

186. B. Because of its tremendous propensity to metastasize, small cell carcinoma is generally considered to have spread to distant sites by the time of diagnosis. Mediastinoscopy with biopsy and, if negative, subsequent thoracotomy for cure, would, thus, not be indicated. However, the staging procedures listed in B are useful because patients with clinically manifest disease limited to one hemithorax and regional nodes (limited stage disease) have a better prognosis with therapy than patients with disease beyond this (extensive stage disease). (Ref. 1, pp. 1118, 1119)

187. D. The chest radiograph in Figure 2.34 reveals bilateral hilar and right paratracheal adenopathy due to sarcoidosis. While most characteristic of sarcoidosis, this radiographic presentation may be seen with fungal and tuberculous infections and with lymphomas. Metastatic ovarian adenocarcinoma would more likely present with pleural effusion and/or parenchymal lung nodules. (Ref. 16, p. 620)

188. C. In the absence of palpable lymph nodes or cutaneous lesions, transbronchial biopsy via the flexible fiberoptic bronchoscope is the initial method of choice to establish a diagnosis of intrathoracic sarcoidosis. Sixty percent of sarcoid patients with radiographic bilateral hilar adenopathy and clear lung fields will show parenchymal granulomas on transbronchial biopsy. While the yield of granulomas is higher with both mediastinoscopy and open lung biopsy, so is the risk to the patient. SACE levels lack both sensitivity and specificity for diagnosis but may be useful in following the clinical course of sarcoidosis patients. Reliable Kveim-Siltzbach antigen is not generally available. (Ref. 1, p. 1450)

189. E. Arthritis and erythema nodosum due to sarcoidosis ("Lofgren's syndrome") generally resolve spontaneously within several months of onset and can be adequately controlled with nonsteroidal antiinflammatory agents. Myocardial involvement with arrhythmias or heart failure, ocular involvement with uveitis, progressive pulmonary disease, and significant central nervous system involvement of various types require systemic corticosteroids. (Ref. 1, pp. 1447–1450)

190. E. The ECG in Figure 2.35 demonstrates a short ($\leq$0.12 seconds) PR interval of 0.08 seconds, a slur on the upstroke of the QRS interval (delta wave), and a prolonged ($\geq$0.12 seconds) QRS complex of 0.15 seconds. These are the characteristic changes of the Wolff-Parkinson-White (WPW) syndrome, a form of ventricular preexcitation due to an AV nodal bypass tract. From 10% to 36% of patients with ventricular preexcitation have supraventricular arrhythmias. Of these, 80% have PSVT, 15%–30% have atrial fibrillation, and 5% have atrial flutter; rarely, the latter two arrhythmias may have extremely rapid ventricular rates sufficient to produce hypotension or sudden death. A few patients have ventricular tachycardia or sinus node dysfunction, while many have no arrhythmias. (Ref. 9, pp. 202, 203, 691)

191. B. All of the maneuvers listed, except hyperventilation, enhance vagotonia, which may terminate PSVT associated with AV-node reentry. (Ref. 9, p. 682)

192. E. Digoxin, verapamil, propranolol, and type 1 antiarrhythmics such as quinidine may be efficacious in preventing PSVT. Lidocaine is useful for ventricular but not supraventricular arrhythmias. (Ref. 9, pp. 682, 683)

193. B. Of patients with WPW, 15%–30% experience intermittent atrial fibrillation. Digoxin, verapamil, and lidocaine may all increase the ventricular rate during atrial fibrillation in these patients and should be avoided as single therapeutic agents. Type 1 antiarrhythmics (quinidine, disopyramide, and procainamide) and amiodarone do not increase the ventricular rate during atrial fibrillation and may provide useful prophylaxis of PSVT in WPW patients. (Ref. 9, pp. 638, 691, 692)

194. E. The clinical signs and symptoms of PE are not sufficiently sensitive or specific to rule in or rule out the diagnosis of PE. Less than one half of patients with PE have clinical evidence of deep vein thrombosis of the lower extremities. While most patients with PE have some kind of abnormality of the chest radiograph (eg, elevated hemidiaphragm, infiltrate, pleural effusion, or zone of hyperlucency), a significant proportion of patients have a normal study. Up to 13% of patients with PE have an arterial PaO_2 greater than 80 torr; a normal PaO_2 does not exclude PE. Only patients with extensive embolization and pulmonary hypertension have ECG evidence of right ventricular strain; most patients have a normal ECG aside from sinus tachycardia. (Ref. 1, pp. 1107, 1108; Ref. 2, pp. 444, 445)

195. B. Patients with low probability V/Q scans, but with a reasonable to high suspicion for PE on the basis of clinical findings and laboratory tests, should undergo pulmonary angiography; up to 10% or more of these patients will prove to have PE. Similarly, since 10%–15% of patients with high probability V/Q scans have negative pulmonary angiograms, these patients should also have angiography if they are at higher than average risk of hemorrhage with anticoagulant therapy. Unless there are contraindications, patients with indeterminate V/Q scans require angiography; 20%–30% prove to have PE. (Ref. 2, pp. 444–447)

196. E. The optimal prothrombin time for long-term anticoagulation of PE patients is 1.2–1.5 times the control (14–17 seconds); this degree of anticoagulation is as effective as a PT of 1.5–2.0 times control and is associated with a four-fold lower rate of hemorrhagic complications. Thrombolytic agents do not improve mortality or pulmonary perfusion any more than heparin in patients with submassive PE but carry a higher bleeding risk. Concurrent administration of antiplatelet agents increases the risk of bleeding during heparin therapy. Heparin therapy may result in significant thrombocytopenia, and serial monitoring of the platelet count is necessary. The full antithrombotic efficacy of warfarin does not occur until after 4–5 days of administration, thereby necessitating this period of overlap with heparin therapy. (Ref. 2, pp. 447–449)

197. B. Low dose subcutaneous heparin does not adequately prevent venous thromboembolism in patients who undergo hip surgery; these patients require warfarin to a prothrombin time of 1.2–1.5 times control, higher doses of subcutaneous heparin, or external pneumatic compression. It is also not effective for patients undergoing surgery for gynecologic malignancies. Low dose heparin is contraindicated in patients undergoing ophthalmic or central nervous system surgery and in spinal cord trauma patients. (Ref. 2, pp. 386, 449)

198. D. The clinical picture and ECG findings are consistent with a diagnosis of acute pericarditis. Prinzmetal's or variant angina resulting from coronary artery spasm may cause ST-segment elevation but would not be associated with fever or exacerbation of chest pain in the supine position. Pulmonary embolism and mitral valve prolapse may cause nonspecific ST-segment depression rather than elevation. Dressler's syndrome refers to pericarditis and pleuritis following acute myocardial infarction, an unlikely occurrence in a 25-year-old woman. (Ref. 9, pp. 1360, 1521, 1522)

199. E. Acute pericarditis may be caused by a variety of infectious, autoimmune, and noninfectious etiologies, which do not include sprue. In the outpatient setting, viral or idiopathic acute pericarditis is the most common etiology. (Ref. 9, p. 1488)

200. E. This clinical presentation is consistent with cardiac tamponade from the accumulation of pericardial fluid, making pericardiocentesis the treatment of choice. Diuretic therapy may exacerbate hypotension; instead, administration of IV normal saline may be a useful temporizing measure. Use of an aortic balloon pump or vasodilators, such as nitroprusside, is not clearly beneficial. All forms of anticoagulant or thrombolytic (eg, streptokinase) therapy are contraindicated in patients with pericarditis, as they predispose to pericardial hemorrhage with cardiac tamponade. (Ref. 9, pp. 1492, 1501)

References

1. Petersdorf RG, Adams RD, Braunwald E, et al (eds): *Harrison's Principles of Internal Medicine*, ed 11. New York, McGraw-Hill, 1987.

2. Wyngaarden J, Smith LH Jr (eds): *Cecil Textbook of Medicine*, ed 18. Philadelphia, WB Saunders, 1988.

3. Wintrobe MM, Lee GR, Boggs DR, et al (eds): *Clinical Hematology*, ed 8. Philadelphia, Lea & Febiger, 1981.

4. Wilson JD, Foster DW (eds): *Williams Textbook of Endocrinology*, ed 7. Philadelphia, WB Saunders, 1985.

5. Moschella SL, Hurley HJ (eds): *Dermatology*, ed 2. Philadelphia, WB Saunders, 1985.

6. Rubenstein E, Federman DD (eds): *Scientific American Medicine*. New York, Scientific American, 1983.

7. Rudolf AM, Hoffman JIE (eds): *Pediatrics*, ed 18. Norwalk, CT, Appleton and Lange, 1987.

8. DeVita VT, Hellman S, Rosenberg SA (eds): *Cancer, Principles and Practice of Oncology*, ed 2. Philadelphia, JB Lippincott, 1985.

9. Braunwald E (ed): *Heart Disease—A Textbook of Cardiovascular Medicine*, ed 3. Philadelphia, WB Saunders, 1988.

10. Pritchard JA, MacDonald PC, Gant NF (eds): *Williams Obstetrics*, ed 17. Norwalk, CT, Appleton-Century-Crofts, 1985.

11. Hurst JW (ed): *The Heart*, ed 6. New York, McGraw-Hill, 1986.

12. Rodnan GP, Schumacher HR, Zuaifler NJ (eds): *Primer on the Rheumatic Diseases*, ed 8. Atlanta, Arthritis Foundation, 1983.

13. Kelley WN, Harris ED Jr, Ruddy S, Sledge CB (eds): *Textbook of Rheumatology*, ed 2. Philadelphia, WB Saunders, 1985.

14. McIntyre KM, Lewis AJ (eds): *Textbook of Advanced Cardiac Life Support*. Dallas, American Heart Association, 1981.

15. Sleisenger MH, Fordtran JS (eds): *Gastrointestinal Disease*, ed 3. Philadelphia, WB Saunders, 1983.

16. Guenter CA, Welch MH (eds): *Pulmonary Medicine*, ed 2. Philadelphia, JB Lippincott, 1982.

17. Goldman DR, Brown FH, Levy WK, Slap GB, Sussman EJ (eds): *Medical Care of The Surgical Patient*. Philadelphia, JB Lippincott, 1982.

18. Sabiston DC Jr (ed): *Textbook of Surgery, The Biological Basis of Surgical Practice*, ed 13. Philadelphia, WB Saunders, 1986.

19. Fishman AD (ed): *Pulmonary Diseases and Disorders*. New York, McGraw-Hill, 1980.

20. Montgomery WH, Donegan J, McIntyre KM (eds): 1985 National Conference on standards and guidelines for cardiopulmonary resuscitation and emergency cardiac care. *JAMA* 1986;255:2985–2989.

21. Calkins E, Davis PJ, Ford AB (eds): *The Practice of Geriatrics*. Philadelphia, WB Saunders, 1986.

22. Expert Panel: Report of the National Cholesterol Education Program Expert Panel on detection, evaluation, and treatment of high blood cholesterol in adults. *Arch Intern Med* 1988;148:36–69.

3
Patient Management Problems

Instructions

The objective of the patient management problem is to test the reader's skill and judgment in dealing with patient care situations. These types of problems attempt to place the reader in the position of the clinician and to provide realistic feedback of the consequences of each decision.

A brief history is provided for each patient. After the patient history, a series of management stages is presented (A-1, A-2, etc.). The reader is presented with numerous courses of action or inquiries within each stage and may select a course of action in any sequence within a particular stage.

For each course of action chosen, there are corresponding responses in the response section which begins on page 235. Use the enclosed special pen to reveal the concealed image information. Apply the pen LIGHTLY, from left to right, after the number of the response to visualize the response (which ends at the asterisk*) corresponding to the course(s) of action that were chosen. Utilize the feedback received to determine whether to make additional choices *within* the stage or to move on to the next stage. Once a stage has been left, *do not* go back to it.

The reader is faced with three types of courses of action: those that should be done, those that should be avoided, and those that are optional. The selection of incorrect actions and the failure to select correct actions are both penalized in the scoring system (see p. 181). Optional selections are not penalized.

The individual cases (patients) are classified by the letters A to O. All fifteen should be completed before totaling the score.

The answers and discussions for each case begin on page 182.

Note: To assure full usage of the latent image pen, please recap *tightly* when not in use.

Cardiology

Patrick K. C. Chun, MD

Patient A

A 20-year-old man had a 4-week history of night sweats, malaise, fever, and arthralgia. Physical examination revealed a temperature of 103.5°F, notable swelling of his right wrist and left ankle, and pain on motion. There were petechiae present on his palms, soles, and in the conjunctiva. There were no abnormal cardiovascular findings on auscultation. His temperature continued to spike in spite of the fact that he was given high doses of IV penicillin.

A-1. Your first step(s) would be to

1. inquire as to a history of drug abuse
2. perform a biopsy of a petechial lesion
3. inquire as to a history of rheumatic fever
4. inquire as to a history of venereal contact
5. obtain an orthopedic evaluation
6. perform a lumbar puncture

A-2.

7. obtain blood cultures
8. obtain urine cultures
9. perform a bone marrow aspiration and biopsy
10. perform a total body CT scan
11. obtain a ventilation-perfusion scan
12. obtain a pulmonary arteriogram

A-3. Your next step(s) would be to
13. aspirate the wrist and ankle
14. perform a thoracentesis and pleural biopsy
15. reexamine the patient
16. obtain a chest x-ray
17. obtain an HLA-B27
18. obtain a lupus preparation

A-4. In addition, one would obtain
19. an echocardiogram
20. skull x-rays
21. a liver-spleen scan
22. a multigated acquisition study
23. a first-pass equilibrium study
24. an aortogram

A-5. To confirm the findings, one should then
25. order an electroencephalogram (EEG)
26. order a brain scan
27. perform a cardiac catheterization
28. perform a liver biopsy
29. Holten monitor the patient
30. order a vectorcardiogram

A-6. Treatment should include
31. changing antibiotics
32. stat IV digitalis
33. thoracic surgery consultation
34. Swan-Ganz catheterization monitoring in the CCU
35. stat IV nitroprusside
36. stat bolus of diazoxide

Thc patient remains stable for about 2 weeks but is later found to be in acute pulmonary edema.

A-7. Step(s) should now include
37. reexamination of the patient
38. CT scan of the heart
39. treadmilling the patient
40. fluoroscopy of the heart
41. Doppler of the heart
42. repeat cardiac catheterization (see Figure 3.1)
43. reecho heart

A-8. Treatment should now include
44. thoracic surgery consultation
45. nephrology consultation
46. upper GI series
47. barium enema
48. barium swallow
49. cardiac series

The patient did well until the morning prior to discharge from the hospital, when he had acute onset of dyspnea, tachycardia, and hypotension.

Figure 3.1

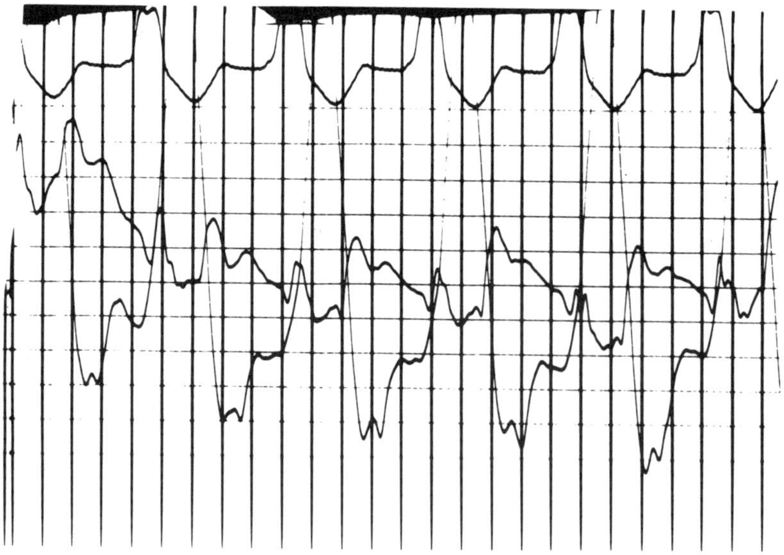

A-9. What step(s) would you take now?

50. Order a stat pulmonary arteriogram
51. Order a stat cerebral arteriogram
52. Order a stat ventilation-perfusion scan
53. Perform a thallium treadmill test
54. Order a technetium pyrophosphate scan
55. Reexamine the patient

A-10. To confirm your findings, you will request which of the following?

56. ECG
57. Chest x-ray (see Figure 3.2)
58. Echocardiogram (see Figure 3.3)
59. Fluoroscopy of the heart (see Figure 3.4)
60. Repeat cardiac catheterization (see Figure 3.5)
61. Thoracic surgery consultation

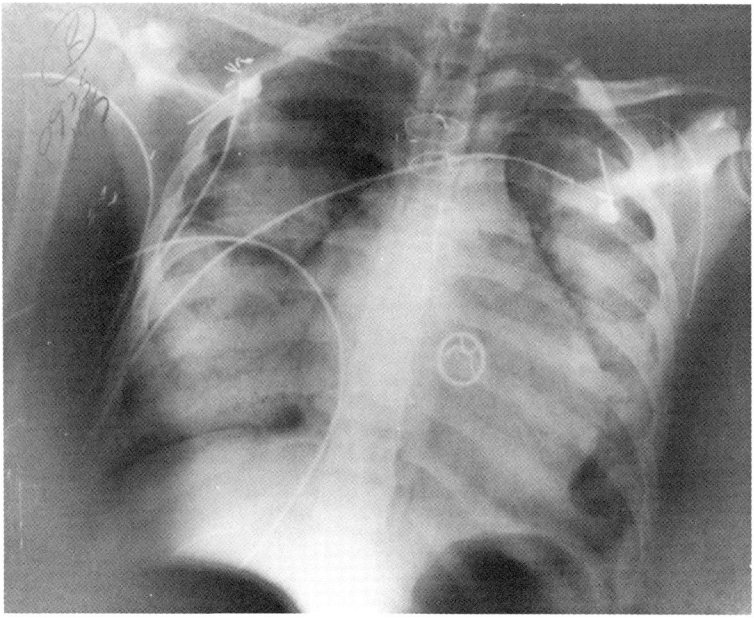

Figure 3.2

Figure 3.3

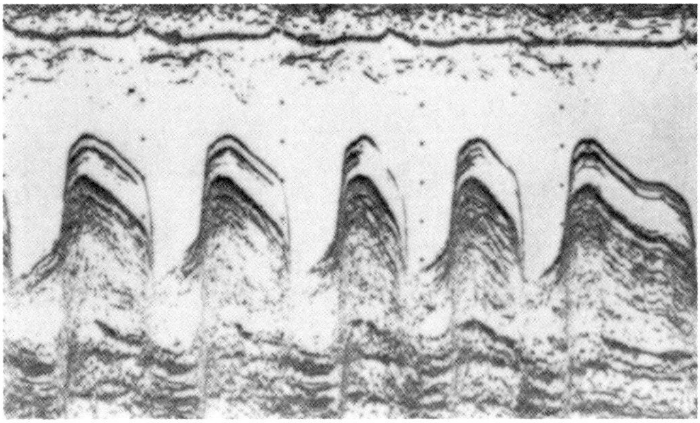

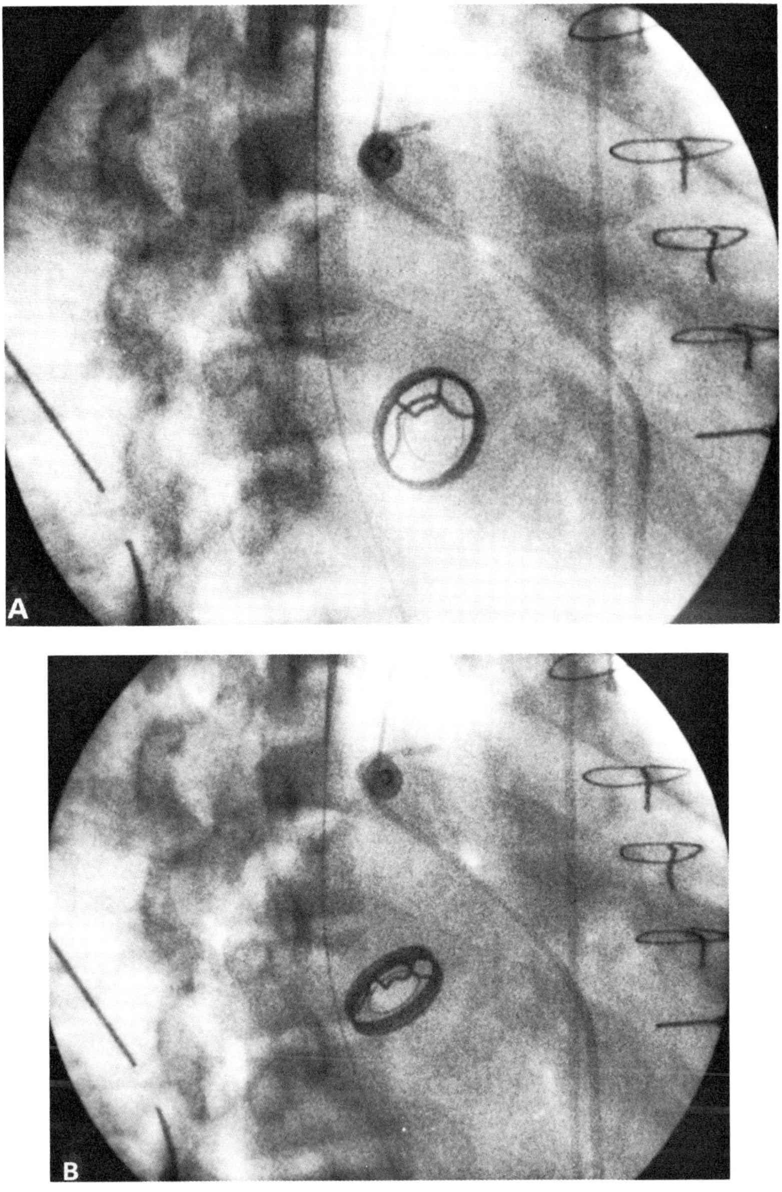

Figure 3.4

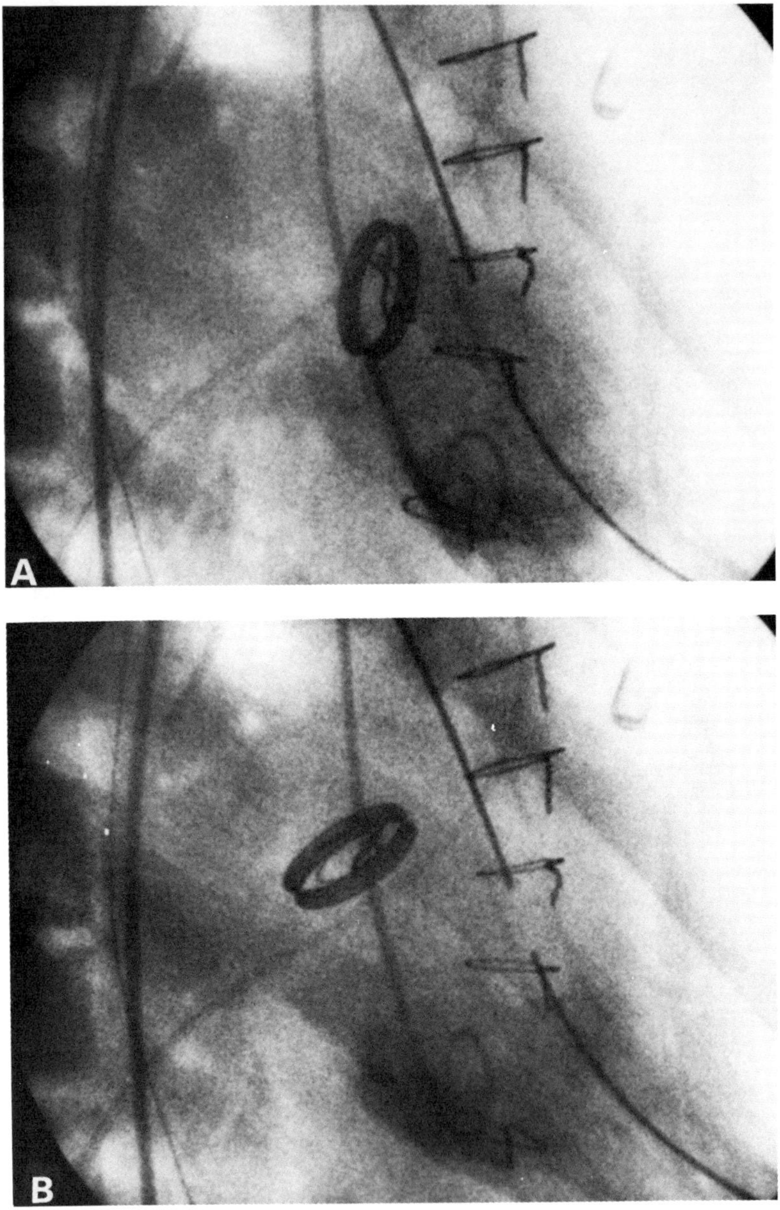

Figure 3.5

Dermatology

William P. Coleman III, MD

Patient B

A 42-year-old woman presents with a 6-month history of a rash of the arms, legs, back, and chest and a flaking scalp. See Figures 3.6 and 3.7.

B-1. Additional history should include which of the following?

1. Any family history of similar problems
2. Any itching of lesions
3. Any medications being taken by patient
4. Is problem worse in winter
5. Any hair loss
6. Any joint pain

B-2. Physical examination should include

7. scalp
8. mouth
9. eyes
10. ears
11. hands
12. genitalia
13. back

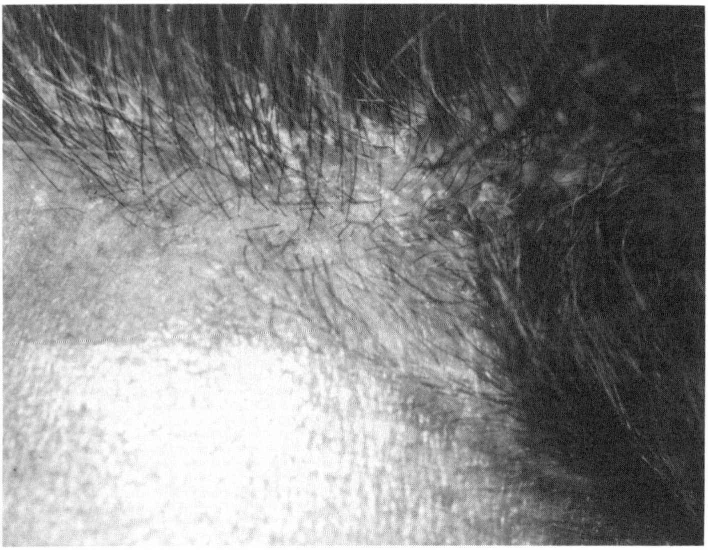

Figure 3.6

B-3. Appropriate initial laboratory tests include

14. CBC (complete blood count)
15. ANA (antinuclear antibodies)
16. bacterial culture of tongue lesions
17. fungal culture of nails
18. bacterial culture of scalp lesions
19. KOH (potassium hydroxide) preparation of genitalia lesion scrapings
20. KOH of sacral lesion scrapings

B-4. Additional laboratory tests and/or special procedures needed include

21. KOH of scalp scrapings
22. chest x-ray
23. gynecological consult
24. hand x-ray
25. draw HLA-antigen studies
26. biopsy for immunofluorescence
27. biopsy for H&E (hematoxylin and eosin)

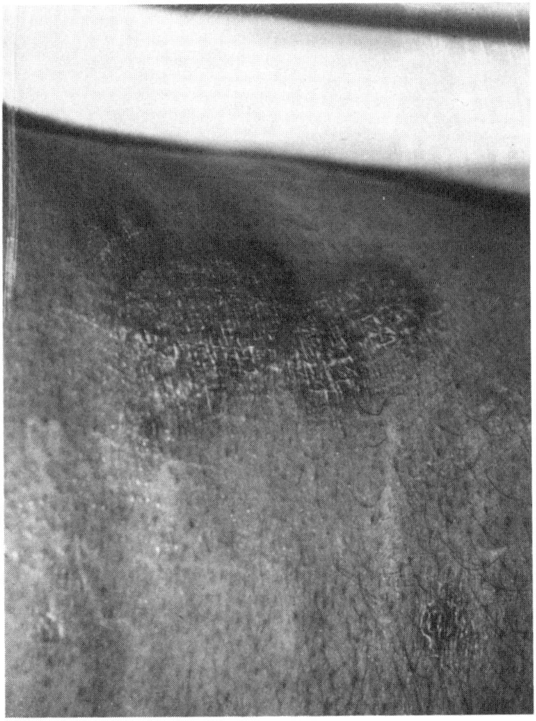

Figure 3.7

B-5. Diagnosis
28. Pityriasis rosea
29. Lupus erythematosus
30. Seborrheic dermatitis
31. Lichen planus
32. Psoriasis
33. Rheumatoid arthritis

B-6. Correct therapy and management include
34. IM triamcinolone 80 mg
35. daily tar shampoos
36. vigorous scrubbing with washcloth in the bath
37. topical hydrocortisone
38. topical fluocinonide
39. tar bath oils
40. ultraviolet light exposure

Gastroenterology

William A. Sodeman, Jr., MD

Patient C

You are the attending physician on the student health service at a major midwestern university. Although the student health service is small, you have the entire resources of the university medical center to draw on.

The patient in question is a 21-year-old white graduate student. She presents with a history of feeling "poorly" for the past several days. She really came to the clinic because she awoke for the second morning in a row with the feeling of pain and stiffness in both hands and today with some discomfort in the right knee. This is her first visit to the student health service. A self-completed history done at the time of application to graduate school contains no history of prior illness.

C-1. Additional history should include which of the following courses of action?

1. Inquire concerning a recent URI (upper respiratory infection), rash, or other infection
2. Inquire concerning hematuria or other urinary tract complaints
3. Seek a history of rash
4. Inquire concerning the development of similar complaints among roommates or close associates
5. Elicit a careful history of drug and medication use in the last 6 weeks
6. Inquire concerning exposure to chemical compounds or toxic agents either at home or within the context of the classroom

Pain and stiffness involving the proximal interphalangeal (PIP) joints of both hands occurred for the first time on the morning of the day prior to coming to the clinic. This recurred on the morning of the clinic visit. The stiffness subsided after an hour or so. On the day of the visit, the patient noted pain in the right knee with some puffiness. There is no history of bone or joint complaints in the past. Specifically, there is no history of rheumatic fever or "growing pains" as a child. The only family history of arthritis involves her father, who suffered a torn ligament in his left knee secondary to trauma.

Physical examination revealed no redness, heat, or deformity in the PIP joints of either hand. There seemed to be no restriction of motion in the fingers. Grip seemed weakened. The right knee was warm to touch and small effusion was present.

C-2. Additional points of importance to check for during the physical exam include

7. rash
8. subcutaneous tissue
9. ophthalmologic exam
10. neurologic exam
11. palpable thyroid
12. rectal exam with test for occult blood

C-3. Initial laboratory tests should include
13. CBC
14. urinalysis
15. latex and ANA
16. antistreptolysin O
17. chest x-ray
18. ECG
19. SMA (sequential multichannel autoanalyzer) 12

C-4. Because of the results of the above tests, coupled with the abnormality of bilirubin and liver-related enzymes, the diagnostic effort should refocus to include
20. HbsAg
21. anti-HBe
22. anti-HBc
23. liver biopsy
24. monospot

The patient appears to have acute viral hepatitis type B. The patient is a single woman who shares a two-bedroom apartment with another student. She has a single boyfriend with whom she has been sexually active, but he does not "live in." She is enrolled in two classes and one seminar and serves as a teaching assistant in a language laboratory course.

C-5. Which of the following management actions are in order?
25. Immediate hospitalization with bed rest and bathroom privileges until bilirubin begins to fall
26. Weekly SGOT (serum glutamic-oxaloacetic transaminase) and bilirubin
27. Hepatitis B immune globulin (HBIG) for her roommate and boyfriend
28. HBIG prophylaxis for classmates and students

You have followed the patient for 6 months since the onset of clinical symptoms. She is still ill, both clinically as well as biochemically. She has taken a leave from the graduate program and moved back with her parents. She is pressing for answers. It is clearly time for a reassessment.

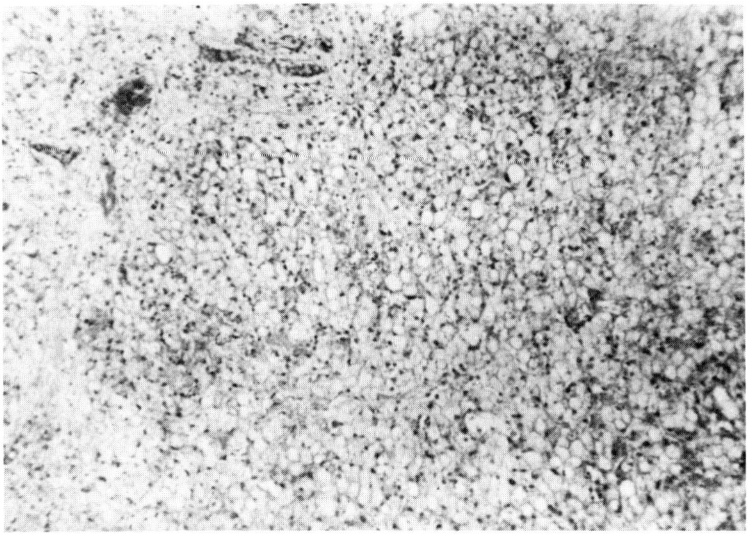

Figure 3.8. Photomicrograph of liver biopsy.

C-6. You do which of the following?

29. HBsAg, anti-HBe, and anti-HBc
30. Liver biopsy (see Figure 3.8)
31. Start prednisone in dose of 60 mg daily
32. Return her to full activity

Nephrology

Alvin E. Parrish, MD

Patient D

A 46-year-old woman is admitted through the emergency room with a complaint of fever, chills, and shaking. She gives a history of having diabetes mellitus that has been controlled with moderate doses of insulin and diet since the age of 14. Her present symptoms began 2 weeks earlier with burning on and frequency of urination. This was followed by lower abdominal pain, dull in nature, and anorexia. One week ago she began to have a fever (100°F). She was treated with a sulfonamide, but in spite of this, her symptoms worsened and the morning of admission to the hospital she developed shaking chills and a high fever.

She has a strong family history of diabetes but no other known diseases. As a child, she had repeated episodes of cystitis and was told that she would outgrow it.

Physical Examination

Her findings were BP 165/95; P 105; R 23; T 103.5°F; Wt 150 lb. She was a well-developed woman in moderate distress. The only other abnormal physical findings were tenderness to palpation over her lower abdomen, bilateral flank and costovertebral angle tenderness, and 2+ ankle edema.

D-1. Additional history should include
1. previous antibiotics
2. allergies
3. history of nephritis
4. history of passing kidney stones

D-2. Additional physical examination would include
5. funduscopic examination
6. pelvic examination
7. careful examination of the abdomen
8. examination of her peripheral pulses
9. rectal examination
10. detailed neurologic examination

D-3. Initial laboratory tests would include (see Figure 3.9)
11. blood sugar
12. BUN
13. creatinine
14. CBC
15. serum cholesterol
16. urinalysis
17. urine culture
18. blood culture

D-4. Additional laboratory tests to be done would include
19. CT scan
20. sonography of the abdomen
21. ECG
22. IVP (intravenous pyelogram)
23. renal biopsy
24. chest x-ray

D-5. Diagnosis (see Figure 3.10)
25. Diabetic glomerulosclerosis
26. Nephritis
27. Pyelonephritis
28. Urinary tract infection
29. Interstitial nephritis

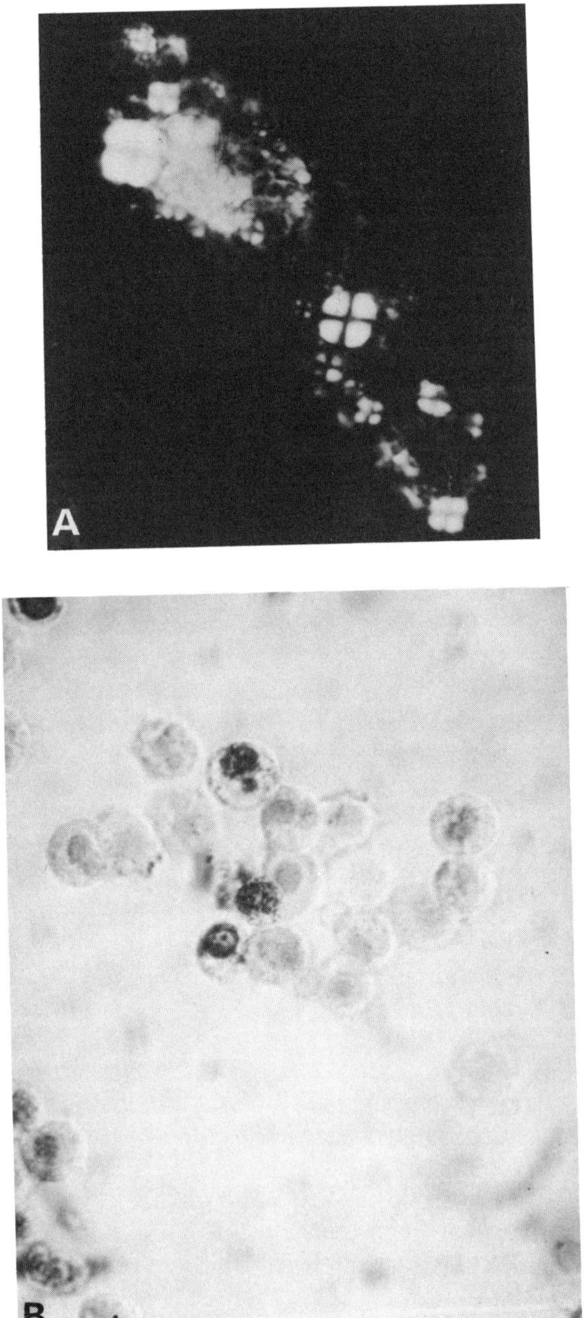

Figure 3.9

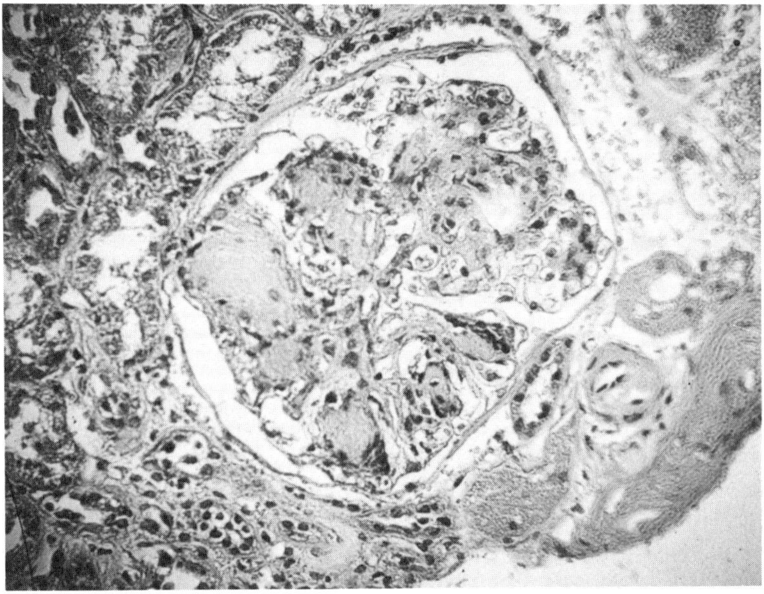

Figure 3.10

D-6. Treatment
30. Increased fluids
31. Ampicillin
32. Tobramycin
33. The appropriate antibiotic depending on the urine culture results and antibiotic sensitivities
34. Antipyretics
35. Cystoscopy with ureteral catheters inserted for proper drainage

She was discharged on an antibiotic, insulin 25 U/d, and a diuretic. Two weeks later she returned with a story of the onset of diarrhea 2 days earlier, amounting to 6 to 8 stools daily. This was accompanied by progressive weakness and lethargy. Examination at this time showed poor skin turgor and a dry mouth. Her BP was 100/60 and fell to 80/50 when she sat up. Other findings were P 100 and T 98.6°F. She appeared acutely ill. There was weakness in her lower extremities, with a decrease in pain sensation in her feet.

D-7. Further history that is necessary includes
36. determination of her dietary intake
37. determination of the approximate volume of her stool
38. determination of her fluid intake
39. history of vomiting
40. current weight

D-8. Additional physical findings would include
41. estimation of degree of hydration
42. rectal exam
43. bowel sounds

D-9. Additional laboratory tests would include
44. CBC
45. urinalysis
46. serum chloride
47. serum sodium
48. serum potassium
49. serum bicarbonate
50. BUN
51. creatinine
52. phosphorous
53. SGOT
54. pH
55. ECG
56. blood volume
57. stool for culture
58. urine culture
59. IVP
60. ultrasound study of abdomen

D-10. Subsequent laboratory studies would include
61. CSF electrolytes
62. renal biopsy

D-11. Diagnosis

63. Chronic renal failure due to diabetic nephropathy
64. Gastroenteritis secondary to antibiotics
65. Acidosis
66. Renal tubular acidosis
67. Bicarbonate-wasting hyperchloremic acidosis
68. Diabetic ketoacidosis
69. Respiratory acidosis
70. Hypochloremic metabolic acidosis

D-12. Treatment

71. Hemodialysis
72. Give 10 g sodium bicarbonate IV
73. Give paregoric or Lomotil®
74. Give a calculated amount of NaCl IV
75. Start IV 5% glucose in water
76. Estimate her fluid and electrolyte losses if any
77. Rapidly rehydrate her with saline
78. Slowly rehydrate her with water

Neurology

William Pryse-Phillips, MD

Patient E

The patient is a 61-year-old carpenter. He complains of moderate headache of 5-months' duration, worse in the last 48 hours, and occurring most days on waking. It usually lasts about 4 to 6 hours and is situated bifrontally with radiation recently to the eyes and neck. The headache is partially relieved by aspirin. His usual physician gave him indomethacin 6 months ago for morning stiffness due to "arthritis," and he has taken it and some white pain killers since that time. Otherwise, he had had only minor complaints such as malaise, mild exertional dyspnea, and a 10-pound weight loss in the last 12 months.

E-1. You might now pause to

1. contact general practitioner for more details
2. arrange for skull x-ray and subsequent CT scan
3. take blood for hematology and ESR
4. administer oxygen 100% for therapeutic trial to relieve current pain
5. instruct clinic nurse to send all medications to pharmacy for identification

E-2. Additional history must include

6. family history of headaches
7. occupational exposure to nitrites
8. ASA allergy
9. prior history of gout
10. prior history of peptic ulcer
11. prior history of sinus disease
12. smoking history

E-3. Further essential subjects for review are

13. dental history
14. muscle stiffness
15. urinary frequency
16. visual disturbances
17. motor power
18. febrile episodes
19. neck pain on movement
20. exertional chest pain

E-4. In your physical examination you would particularly search for

21. carotid bruits
22. joint deformity
23. cervical lymphadenopathy
24. rash
25. scalp tenderness
26. proximal muscle weakness
27. unequal radial pulses
28. diminished visual acuity
29. focal neurologic deficits
30. signs of CO_2 retention
31. fundal venous pulsations
32. fundal hemorrhages
33. orthostatic hypotension

E-5. You notice that the patient's pain is distressing him. Your management step would now be

34. acetaminophen
35. administer 100% oxygen at 7 L/min for migraine
36. attempt headache reduction with amyl nitrite
37. prednisolone 100 mg po
38. prednisolone 10 mg po
39. withhold treatment until the diagnosis is firmly established by laboratory results

E-6. Essential investigations now must include

40. skull, sinus, and cervical spine x-rays
41. isotope brain scan
42. CT scan
43. EEG
44. lumbar puncture
45. serum CK
46. hematology, ESR, electrolytes, BUN

E-7. Which of the following additional studies may be required?

47. Carotid angiography
48. Muscle biopsy
49. Arterial biopsy
50. Liver biopsy
51. Renal biopsy
52. Urinary VMA (vanillylmandelic acid)
53. Serum calcium, phosphate, and alkaline phosphatase
54. Consult ophthalmologist
55. No tests until hematology, ESR, etc., are returned

E-8. Diagnosis

56. Adult-onset migraine
57. Hypertensive headaches
58. Headache secondary to osteoarthritis Cx spine
59. Cranial arteritis
60. Intracranial mass
61. Hydrocephalus ex vacuo secondary to brain atrophy

E-9. Treatment now indicated includes

62. nonsteroidal antiinflammatory drugs, e.g., indomethacin
63. tricyclic analgesics/antidepressants, e.g., amitriptyline
64. high-dose steroids, e.g., prednisone 100 mg/d
65. propranolol 40 mg tid
66. ASA high dosage (1 – 2 g/d) × 18 days

E-10. The prognosis of this condition in a treated case is that the patient

67. is unlikely to survive with intact vision
68. should respond fully with treatment over 1 month
69. should respond fully with treatment over 3 years or more
70. should respond partially with maintained high-dose steroids

Obstetrics and Gynecology

Ralph W. Hale, MD

Patient F

Mrs. Jones is a 32-year-old gravida 4, para 2, abortion 1, who has been your patient for her last two pregnancies. She was first seen by you with the current pregnancy at approximately ten weeks based on her last menstrual period. Her initial examination was consistent with the dates and she is now in her 34th week.

Her prenatal course has been uneventful until one week ago when she was noted to have a slight elevation in blood pressure with 1+ proteinuria (Fig. 3.11). She is now in your emergency room stating that she is having some contractions and she began to bleed about two hours ago. She describes the contractions as mild and the bleeding as bright red enough to soak a pad.

F-1. The following additional history should be obtained

1. a history of recent sexual intercourse
2. previous episodes of bleeding
3. nausea, vomiting, or diarrhea
4. difficulty with voiding
5. change in diet or physical activity
6. alterations in fetal activity
7. history of bleeding in previous pregnancies
8. history of irregular periods

REMINDERS:

G	T	P	A	L	LMP	EDC	INIT.
4	2	2	2	2	January	October 1	

DATE / YEAR	WEIGHT	BLOOD PRESSURE	URINE PROTEIN	URINE SUGAR	EST. WEEKS GESTATION	FUNDAL HEIGHT	POSITION	FHT	EDEMA	RETURN		INIT.
3-12	132	110/59	N	N	10	*		**	0		* Not palpable ** Not heard Hgb 13.2	
4- 8	133¼	108/62	N	N	14	6cm		RLQ 140	0		Spotting after sex	
5- 6	134½	114/68	N	N	18	14cm		RLQ 144	0			
5-27	137	110/60	N	N	21	20cm		LLQ 132	0			
6-20	139	116/64	N	N	24	24cm		LLQ 128	0			
7-10	142	112/58	N	N	28	26cm		RLQ 150	Tr		Hgb 10.8, recommend Fe	
8- 4	146½	118/70	Tr	Tr	31	30cm		RLQ 148	Tr		Rest at home	
8-15	151	128/82	1+	N	33	32cm		RLQ 140	2+		Bed rest, recheck one week	

Figure 3.11

F-2. The initial examination should include

9. blood pressure
10. weight
11. uterine size
12. vaginal speculum examination
13. fetal heart rate
14. cervical consistency and dilation
15. edema

F-3. The initial laboratory tests should include

16. 24-hour urine for protein
17. STAT hemoglobin and hematocrit
18. platelet count
19. fibrinogen levels
20. serum folate
21. urine dipstick

F-4. After the first laboratory findings have been received the following additional tests or procedures should be ordered

22. obstetrical ultrasound (Fig. 3.12)
23. amniocentesis for lung maturity
24. contraction stress test (Fig. 3.13)
25. scalp pH
26. double set up examination

Figure 3.12

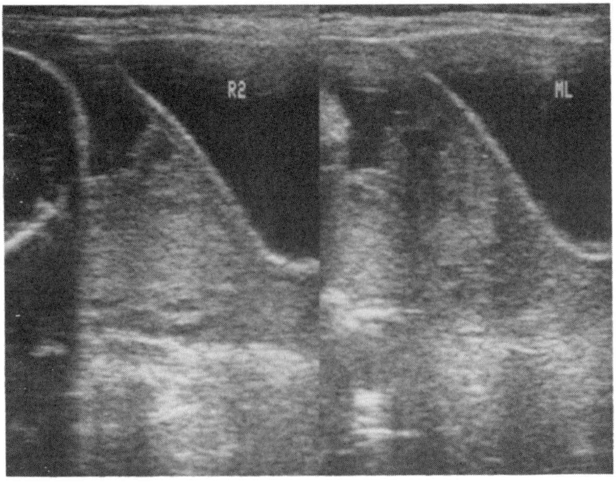

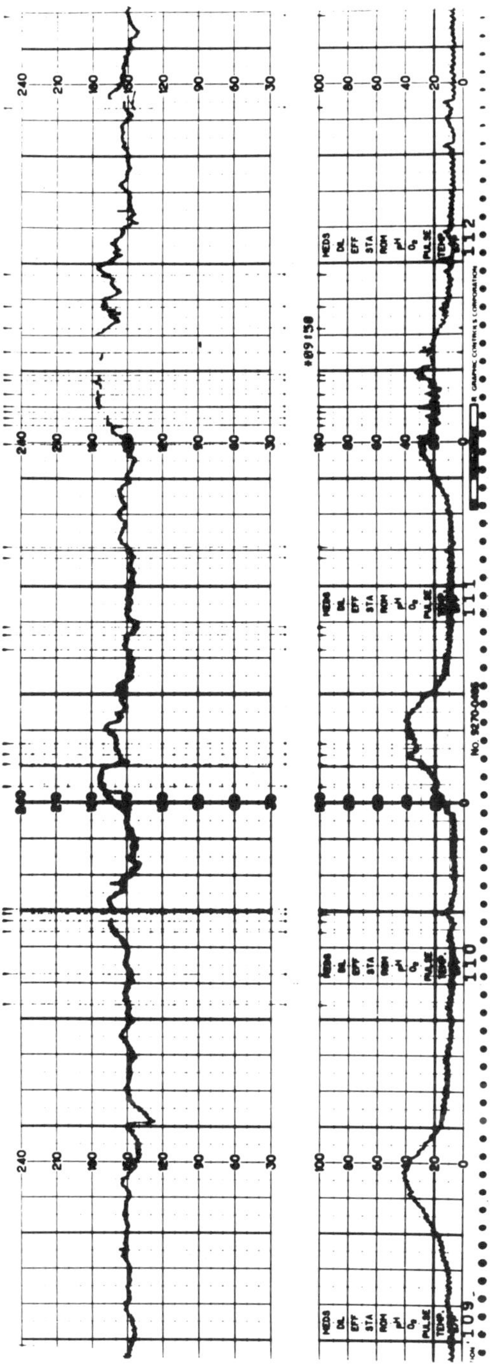

Figure 3.13

F-5. Based on the history, examination, and laboratory findings, the most likely diagnosis is
27. circumvallate placenta
28. premature placental separation
29. placenta previa
30. disseminated intravascular coagulation
31. severe cervicitis

F-6. Therapy and management should include the following courses of action
32. allowing the patient to go home with instructions on bed rest and return if bleeding continues
33. immediate C-section
34. hospitalization and observation
35. transfusion of two units packed cells
36. rupture of the membranes and pitocin induction
37. repeat amniocentesis

Patient G

You are called to the emergency room at 5 PM to evaluate a 19-year-old patient who has just been admitted with a 30-minute history of acute onset of lower right abdominal pain. She relates that it started shortly after she returned home from her last class of the day at the local junior college. She states that it is getting progressively worse. Her vital signs reveal a BP of 90/60, P 96, R 18, T 99.8°F. The abdomen is exquisitely tender with rebound in both lower quadrants. On pelvic examination the cervix is very tender on motion. No masses are palpable. Blood is seen in the cervical os.

G-1. Additional history should include
1. last normal menstrual history
2. sexual history
3. urinary symptoms
4. previous episodes
5. GI symptoms
6. presence of a convulsive disorder

G-2. Additional physical examination should include
7. auscultation of the abdomen
8. evaluation of the costa vertebral angle
9. funduscopic examination
10. evaluation of the deep veins in the leg
11. breast examination
12. chest auscultation

G-3. Initial laboratory tests should include
13. hemoglobin, hematocrit
14. sedimentation rate
15. urine pregnancy test
16. cervical gram stain
17. white blood cell count
18. complete urinalysis

G-4. Additional studies would include (see Figures 3.14 and 3.15)

19. qualitative beta human chorionic gonadotropin (HCG)
20. ultrasonography
21. KUB x-ray
22. urine cultures
23. paracentesis
24. culdocentesis

G-5. Your working diagnosis would be

25. acute appendicitis
26. ectopic pregnancy
27. torsion of an ovarian cyst
28. renal colic
29. Meckel's diverticulum
30. acute salpingitis

Figure 3.14

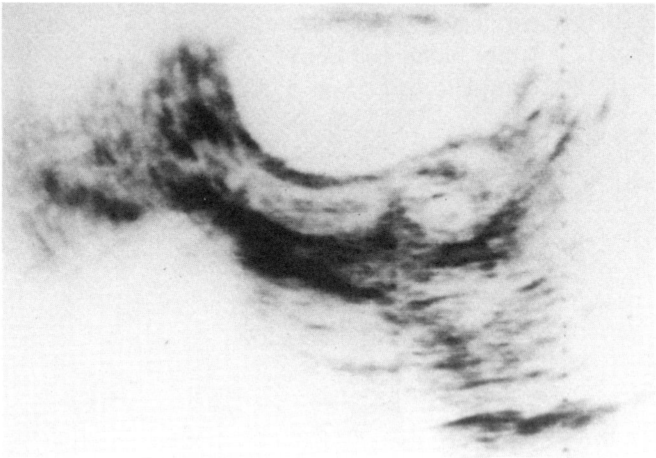

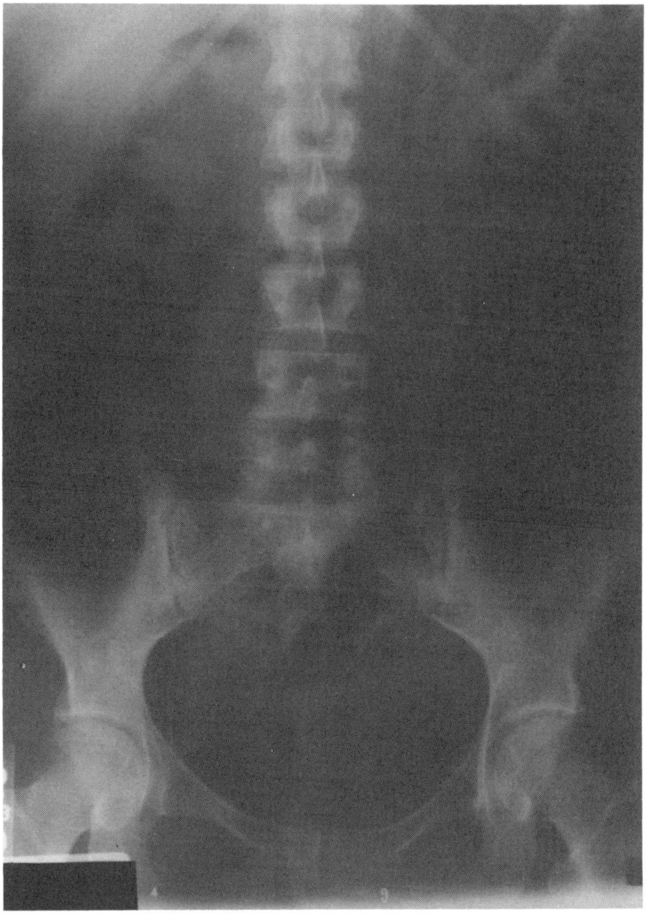

Figure 3.15

G-6. Your immediate treatment should include

31. admission for IV antibiotics and observation
32. discharge on antispasmodics
33. cystoscopy with retrograde pyelography
34. immediate laparotomy
35. laparoscopy
36. transperitoneal aspiration

Patient H

Your patient is a 20-year-old white woman who is at 38 weeks gestation with her first baby. She has had an uneventful prenatal course and is in the office today for her weekly check-up. Your nurse reports that she has gained 8 pounds and has a blood pressure of 150/100. Her urine shows 2+ protein. A review of prenatal records indicates that she had a trace of protein and a blood pressure of 120/70 on her last visit 1 week ago.

H-1. Specific questions that you would ask your patient about include

1. medications
2. vision changes
3. GI symptoms
4. bleeding
5. changes in her life-style
6. alcohol ingestion
7. smoking habits

H-2. Your examination should include which of the following evaluations? (See Figures 3.16 and 3.17).

8. Funduscopic examination
9. X-ray pelvimetry
10. Deep tendon reflexes
11. Cranial nerve assessment
12. Abdominal girth
13. Chest x-ray

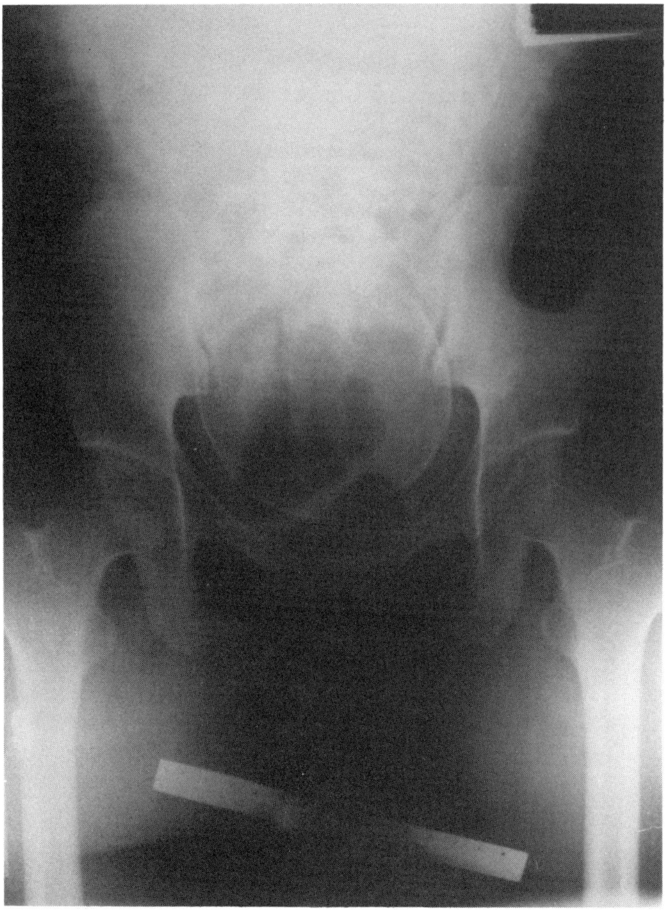

Figure 3.16

H-3. Based on these findings, your initial management should be

14. complete bed rest at home for 48 hours and then reevaluate
15. start furosemide 20 mg po and recheck in 48 hours
16. leave patient in the room for 1 hour and recheck her blood pressure
17. admit to the hospital immediately
18. schedule for induction the following day
19. request a consultation with an internist whose subspecialty is cardiology

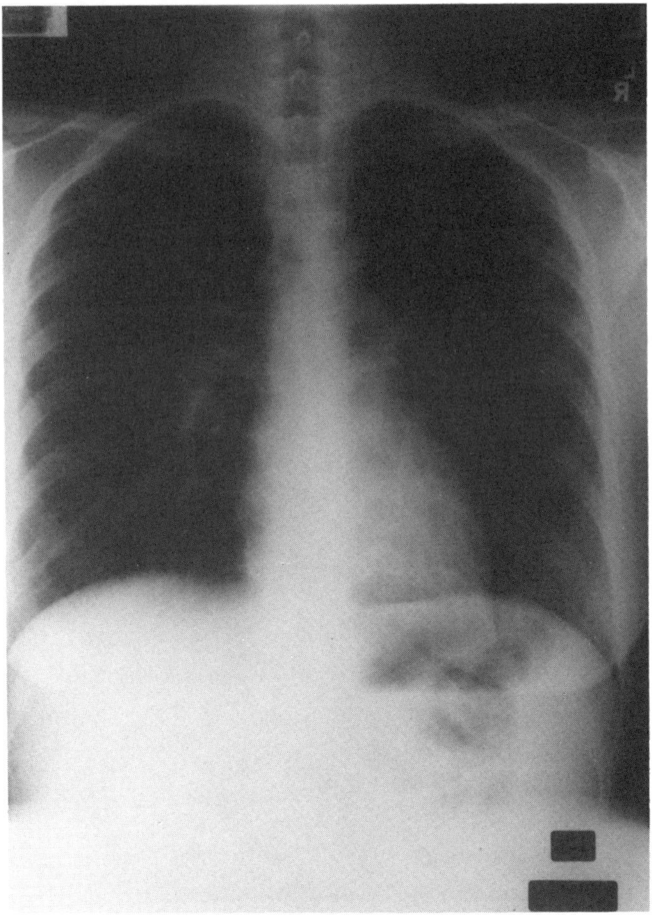

Figure 3.17

H-4. Based on your decision, which of the following laboratory studies should be ordered?

20. Serum calcium and magnesium levels
21. Urinary estriol
22. 24-hour urine protein
23. Creatinine and BUN
24. Serum electrolytes
25. Antinuclear antibodies
26. Platelets
27. Uric acid

H-5. Your working diagnosis is
28. chronic glomerulonephritis
29. severe preeclampsia
30. eclampsia
31. nephrotic syndrome
32. SLE
33. pheochromocytoma

H-6. Appropriate therapy includes
34. immediate cesarean section
35. admission to the hospital for stabilization
36. IV $MgSO_4$
37. carefully controlled induction
38. bed rest at home for 24 to 48 hours
39. diuretic therapy alone

Pediatrics

Victor LaCerva, MD

Patient I

A 15-year-old white girl is brought into the pediatric emergency room. You are the physician in charge. The ambulance driver gives a history of being called to the scene of an accident where the young girl had been struck by a car, falling off of her bicycle and striking the pavement with her head. At the present time, the nurse informs you that the patient is conscious and the vital signs are stable: T 99°F, P 85, R 20, BP 125/85. Her mother has been informed of the accident and should arrive shortly. You enter the examination room and find an apparently well-developed and well-nourished girl who is anxious but otherwise in no distress. She has an obvious abrasion on her left forehead, which the nurse is cleaning.

I-1. You begin to expand on the history you already have, with particular emphasis on which of the following?

1. Circumstances of the accident
2. Loss of consciousness at the time of the accident
3. Complaints at the present time
4. Past history of hospitalizations
5. Past history of allergies
6. History of drug or alcohol abuse
7. Family and social history
8. Review of systems

I-2. You proceed with a physical examination, paying special attention to which of the following areas?

9. Neurologic evaluation
10. HEENT and neck
11. Chest and cardiovascular systems
12. Abdominal exam
13. Rectal exam
14. Inspection of the genitalia
15. Range of motion of all joints
16. Examination of the skin for bruises, lacerations, or signs of injury

I-3. In view of the history and findings on physical exam, you proceed with which of the following laboratory tests?

17. CBC
18. Urinalysis
19. ECG
20. Skull x-ray
21. Abdominal flat and upright x-rays
22. Chest x-ray (see Figure 3.18)
23. Exam and culture of vaginal discharge

I-4. You are beginning to integrate your history, physical findings, and lab data into a treatment plan. However, you decide that which of the following additional steps are necessary?

24. Repeat vital signs
25. Obtain immunization history
26. Obtain cardiology consult
27. Obtain psychiatric consult
28. Obtain neurologic consult
29. Send blood for type and cross, 2 U
30. Obtain sexual history

I-5. The patient's mother has arrived. You inform her that your work-up is not yet complete. You then proceed to

31. schedule a CT scan
32. obtain a pregnancy test
33. order an IVP stat
34. obtain surgical consult

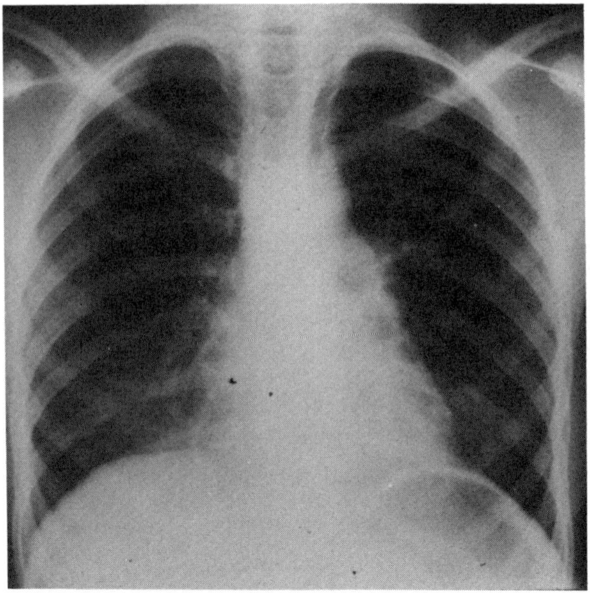

Figure 3.18

I-6. You have arrived at your final decisions and proceed to carry out which of the following?

35. Start an IV line with D5W and observe the patient in the emergency room for at least 2 hours
36. Admit the patient to the hospital for observation overnight
37. Refer to the appropriate clinic
38. Instruct parent and patient on danger signs to look for over the next few days
39. Prescribe topical antibiotics for the abrasion

Patient J

A 17-year-old teenage boy presents in your office with a chief complaint of "burning when I pee." You have known this patient for the past 10 years, but have not seen him in the last 4 years, except once for a sports physical about two years ago. Vital signs are normal.

J-1. You begin by asking how he has been in general, ("fine"), and then proceed to take a more detailed history, paying special attention to

1. a review of his immunization status
2. any known allergies
3. general review of systems
4. past history of hospitalizations
5. "How are you doing in school?"
6. "Many young people experiment with cigarettes, alcohol, pot, or other drugs. Have you or your friends ever tried them? What have you tried?"
7. previous history of urinary tract infections
8. duration and degree of present symptoms
9. medications taken for present illness
10. sexual orientation
11. past sexual partners
12. details of kind of sexual activity

J-2. He appears to be in good general physical condition. You perform an exam, paying special attention to which of the following points?

13. HEENT (head, eyes, ears, nose, and throat)
14. Fundoscopic exam
15. Joint mobility
16. CVA tenderness
17. Auscultation of chest and heart
18. Examination of the testicles
19. Examination of the penis
20. Rectal exam

J-3. You decide to order a number of laboratory tests. These include

21. complete blood count (CBC)
22. SMA 6 (electrolytes, glucose, BUN)
23. blood cholesterol
24. chest x-ray
25. urinalysis
26. urine culture and sensitivity
27. scraping of penile lesion
28. gram stain of urethral discharge
29. gonorrhea culture of urethral discharge
30. microtrac exam for chlamydia on penile discharge
31. gonorrhea culture of throat
32. gonorrhea culture of rectum
33. HIV antibody test

J-4. To confirm your diagnosis at this point you would

34. consult with a psychiatrist
35. refer for a darkfield examination
36. do a punch biopsy of the penile lesion
37. do a rapid plasma reagin (RPR) test for syphilis
38. review gram stain of urethral discharge
39. do Tzanck prep of scraping from penile lesion

J-5. As a result of all the information you have so far, you would

40. treat with benzathine penicillin G 2.4 million units IM
41. treat with aqueous procaine penicillin G 4.8 million units IM plus probenecid 1.0 gram by mouth, followed by tetracycline 500 mg qid for 1 week
42. treat with tetracycline 500 mg qid for 1 week alone
43. apply podophyllin in benzoin to the penile lesion
44. provide condoms
45. reschedule for a return visit and test of cure
46. provide safer sex counseling
47. recommend that sexual partners be evaluated and treated

J-6. The patient returns 4 days after completion of therapy. He is free of symptoms. His present girlfriend has been evaluated and treated. His urethral gonorrhea culture was positive, as was his HIV test. Further management at this time includes

48. PPD
49. RPR for syphilis if not already done
50. test of cure culture
51. refer sexual partners for HIV testing
52. refer close coworkers for HIV testing
53. start IgG treatments monthly
54. refer to doctor knowledgeable about AIDS
55. examine for presence of enlarged lymph nodes
56. review precautions necessary to avoid exposing loved ones
57. discuss poor prognosis
58. review signs and symptoms of AIDS

Patient K

Baby Ruth presents in your office at 1 month of age with a chief complaint of a stuffy nose. The mother is tired looking and appears to be quite anxious about the health of her daughter. The infant visited another physician at about 1 week of age because of jaundice and feeding problems. The mother has been reassured by friends and relatives that the baby is probably fine, but she remains concerned. As you undress the baby for height and weight, you begin to share her concern. The infant appears quite undernourished. You proceed to take a history before beginning your examination of the infant.

K-1. You begin taking your history, paying special attention to

1. problems during pregnancy
2. birth weight
3. birth history
4. neonatal course
5. problems with jaundice
6. feeding history
7. health of siblings
8. occupation of the father
9. suspicions of retardation in this infant
10. history of previous doctor visit

K-2. You begin your exam, focusing on which of the following aspects?

11. Minor congenital anomalies
12. Development
13. Size of the fontanelles
14. Cardiovascular system
15. Abdominal exam
16. Neurologic status
17. Hip range of motion
18. Vaginal exam with nasal speculum
19. Examination of the skin

K-3. You begin to write orders for certain lab tests to be done. These include

20. CBC
21. urinalysis
22. urine culture
23. urine for 17-ketosteroids
24. chest x-ray
25. ECG
26. bilirubin studies
27. liver function studies
28. chromosome studies
29. TORCH studies
30. thyroid studies
31. plot data on growth curve

K-4. To further confirm your suspected diagnosis, you would

32. consult with a neurologist
33. discuss with the mother hospitalizing the infant for additional work-up
34. review the hospital birth record to seek diagnostic clues
35. take a more detailed feeding history
36. inquire about the use of breastfeeding devices
37. observe a feeding
38. inquire about maternal diet and her level of fatigue
39. proceed with a sepsis work-up

K-5. Management of the case now consists of

40. referral to a developmental specialist
41. bottle feeding a formula with iron
42. giving appropriate breastfeeding counseling
43. rescheduling a visit in 1 week
44. prescription for maternal rest and relaxation
45. begin thyroxine therapy
46. begin multivitamins for the infant

Psychiatry

Barbara Ann Allen, PhD, and
James R. Allen, PhD

Patient L

A 22-year-old college student is brought to the emergency room by his roommate and dormitory counsellor. They state the young man has always been somewhat of an isolate but had become much more withdrawn and suspicious over the last 3 or 4 weeks. He stopped going to classes 1 week ago and locked himself in his room, allowing only his roommate to come in. For the past 3 days he has refused to eat and has begun to talk of vague plots against him. Today, he accused his roommate of being in league with his enemies.

L-1. Your first step would be to

1. give antipsychotic medication IM stat since the patient obviously is psychotic
2. interview and examine the patient
3. sign commitment forms
4. obtain blood and urine for a drug screen

L-2. You would also want to know which of the following?

5. Recent stressors
6. History of previous episodes of a similar nature
7. Family history of schizophrenic disorder
8. History of drug abuse
9. History of past health and current medications
10. Family history of bipolar disorder
11. CT scan abnormalities

L-3. In the mental status examination, you would be particularly interested in eliciting which of the following?

12. Auditory hallucinations
13. Delusions
14. Thought insertion
15. Thought broadcasting
16. Hypochondriasis
17. History of headaches

L-4. Your next step would be to select which of the following?

18. Physical examination
19. Drug screen
20. CT scan
21. Urinary 3,4 MHPG
22. CSF 50-HIAA (5-hydroxyindoleacetic acid)

L-5. Which of the following would be important in establishing a diagnosis for this man?

23. History of marked psychosocial stress; illness less than 2 weeks
24. Decline in functioning for more than 6 months
25. Relationship with his father
26. Family history of schizophrenic disorder or mania
27. Negative symptoms of schizophrenic disorder

L-6. The most likely diagnosis for this young man is

28. schizophreniform disorder
29. bipolar disorder, manic
30. factitious psychological disorder
31. schizoaffective disorder

L-7. Your next step would be to
32. give haloperidol 5 mg stat
33. give imipramine 50 mg IM stat
34. give Librium 24 mg IM stat

L-8. The first evening in the hospital, the patient developed a sudden, painful contraction of his left sternocleidomastoid muscle. This is an example of
35. acute dystonia
36. a basal ganglia side effect
37. akinesia
38. parkinsonian syndrome

L-9. The most appropriate treatment is
39. Congentin 2 mg IM
40. Haldol 5 mg IM
41. a sedative-type antipsychotic
42. an analgesic

On the third day after admission, the patient is much improved. He says he no longer is hearing voices, and he has begun to socialize with the other patients.

A very energetic third-year medical student orders a DST. The initial 8 AM value of cortisol is in the high-normal range and it does decrease by the next morning following the administration of 1 mg dexamethasone at 11 PM.

L-10. This result is most likely
43. an example of suppression
44. an example of nonsuppression
45. a surprise
46. not a surprise

L-11. Which of the following interfere with the DST?
47. Severe weight loss
48. Antidepressant medication
49. Carbamazepine

L-12. Which, if any, of the following EEG tracings is most compatible with the diagnosis of schizophreniform disorder?

50. Figure 3.19
51. Figure 3.20
52. Figure 3.21
53. None of the above

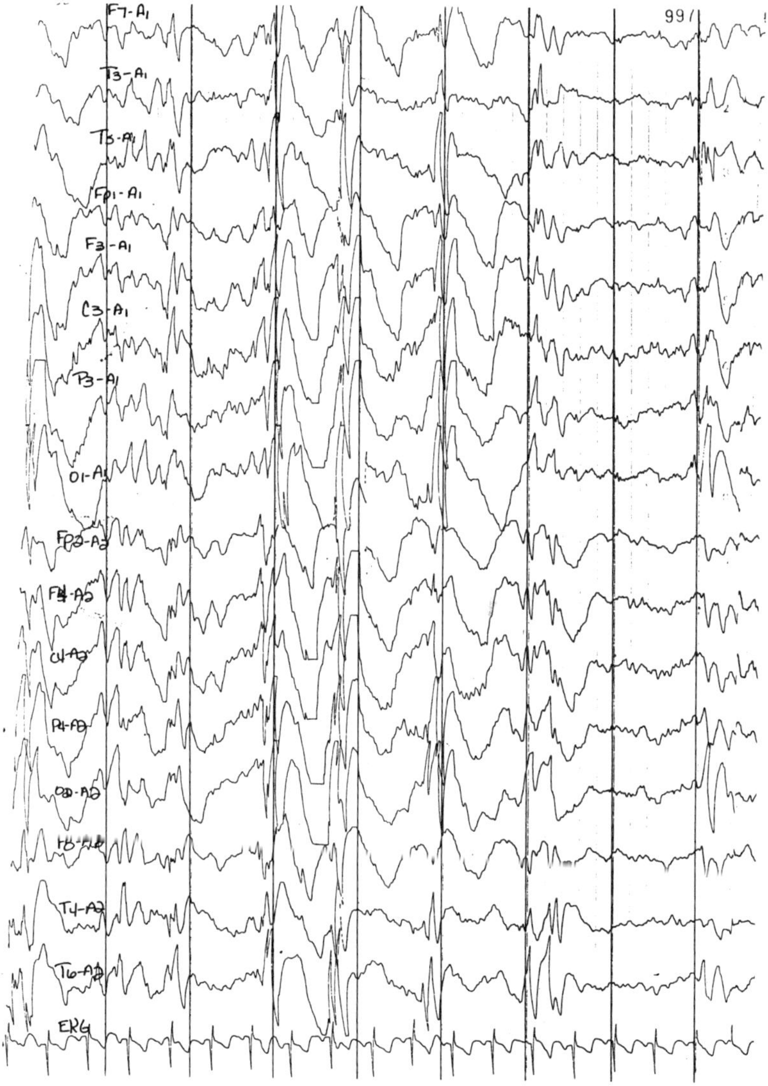

Figure 3.19

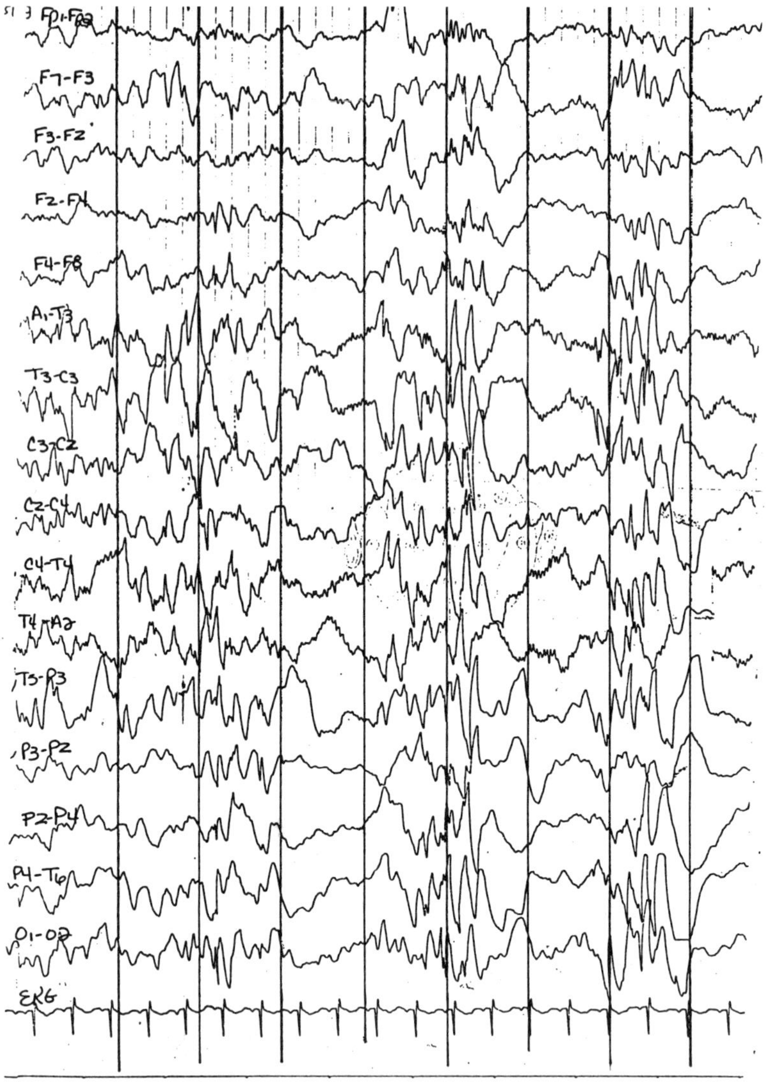
Fp1-Fp2
F7-F3
F3-Fz
Fz-F4
F4-F8
A1-T3
T3-C3
C3-Cz
Cz-C4
C4-T4
T4-A2
T5-P3
P3-Pz
Pz-P4
P4-T6
O1-O2
EKG

Figure 3.20

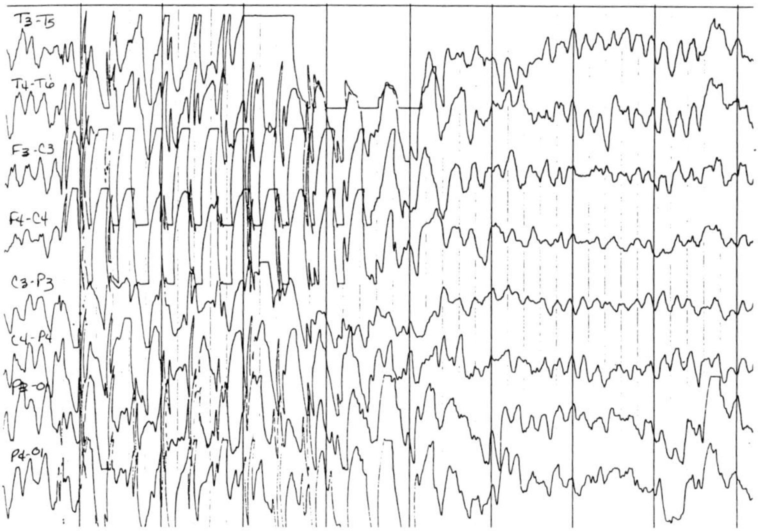

Figure 3.21

Surgery

M. D. Ram, MD

Patient M

A 55-year-old white man was admitted with a history of upper abdominal pain, loss of appetite, and jaundice. He has not been feeling well for over a month and noted that his stool has been light colored on a few occasions. He had an operation about 10 years previously. He dislikes milk and cream products. On occasion, he felt that he had fever but had not documented it. On admission his vital signs were T 100°F, P 66, and BP 140/85 mmHg. For additional information, see Table 3.1.

M-1. Additional history of importance includes

1. blood transfusions
2. drug history
3. history of malaria
4. weight loss
5. details of previous operation
6. alcohol consumption
7. family history

M-2. Clinical evaluation should include

8. abdominal scar
9. abdominal mass
10. ascites
11. rash and scratch marks
12. Murphy's sign
13. stool guaiac
14. caput medusae

TABLE 3.1. Patient M

Test	Result	Normal range
Total bilirubin	9.2	0.1–1.5 mg%
SGOT	65	10–40 U
Serum alkaline phosphatase	350	100–225 U
Total protein	7.2	6.0–8.0 g/dL
Albumin	4.2	3.5–5.0 g/dL

M-3. Laboratory tests should include
15. serum electrolytes
16. liver profile
17. hemogram
18. urine urobilinogen
19. arterial blood gases
20. clotting time (Lee-White)
21. prothrombin time

M-4. Radiologic studies of value are (see Figure 3.22)
22. IV cholangiogram
23. ultrasonography
24. transhepatic cholangiogram
25. superior mesenteric angiogram
26. endoscopic retrograde cholangiopancreatography (ERCP)

M-5. Further steps in management of this patient include
27. blood transfusion
28. IV hyperalimentation
29. parenteral antibiotics
30. oral vitamin supplementation
31. external biliary drainage

M-6. Methods of treatment of the patient include
32. choledochojejunostomy
33. revision of previous anastomosis
34. choledochogastrostomy
35. choledocholithotomy and T-tube drainage
36. hepaticojejunostomy
37. Longmire operation
38. endoscopic papillotomy

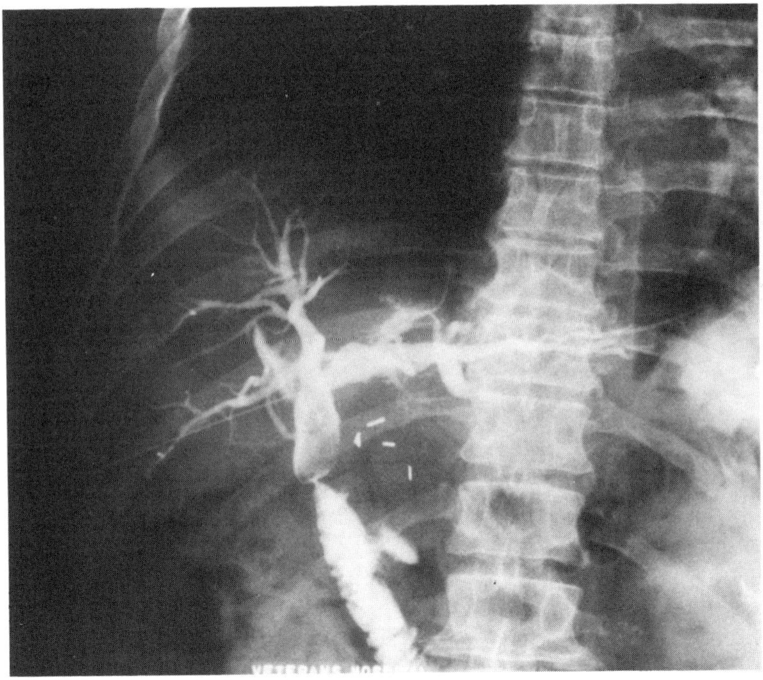

Figure 3.22

Patient N

A 65-year-old obese white man was admitted with lower abdominal colicky pain of 3-days' duration. The pain was in the suprapubic area and in the left lower quadrant. In the past 1 year he had similar pain on three occasions, but it usually resolved in a day or two. He also complained of increasing constipation and episodes of diarrhea for the last 6 months. He has not vomited but feels nauseated and has abdominal distention. He has not passed any stool or gas for 24 hours. On admission his vital signs were T 100.6°F, P 96, BP 150/90 mmHg.

N-1. Additional clinical information required is
1. rectal bleeding
2. laxative usage
3. weight loss
4. urinary problems
5. bowel sounds
6. abdominal mass
7. alcohol intake
8. abdominal tenderness
9. rectal exam

N-2. Initial work-up should include
10. CBC
11. blood culture
12. urine culture
13. stool culture
14. plain abdominal series
15. ultrasound examination of abdomen

N-3. Management of this patient at this stage will include
16. IV fluids
17. parenteral antibiotics
18. oral neomycin and erythromycin
19. bulk laxatives
20. cecostomy
21. frequent vital signs and reevaluation
22. colostomy

N-4. Subsequent studies should include (see Figure 3.23)
23. sigmoidoscopy
24. CT scan
25. IVP
26. cystoscopy
27. cystogram
28. colonoscopy
29. urethrogram

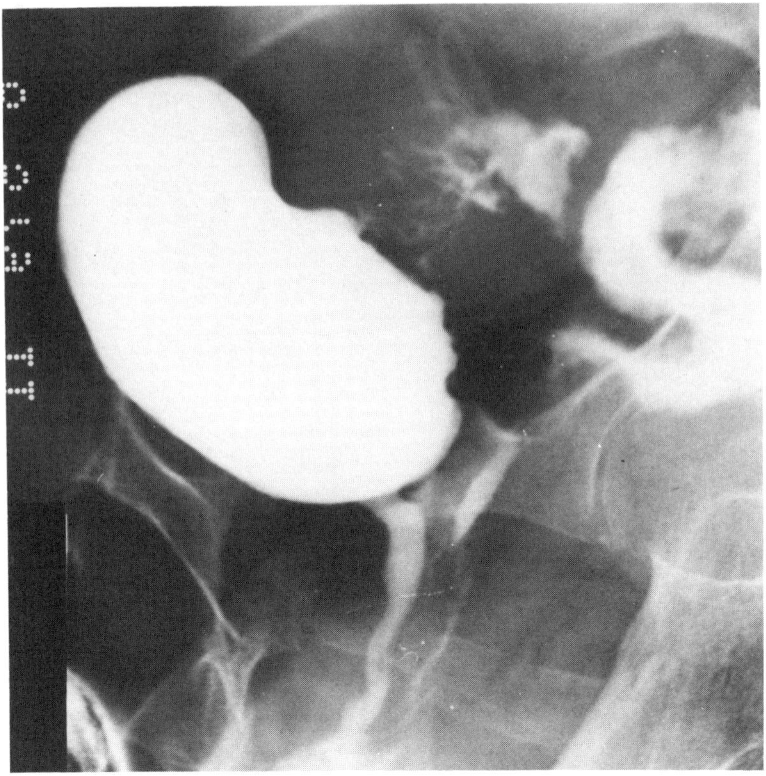

Figure 3.23

N-5. Treatment of the lesion is accomplished by

30. primary resection of colon, repair of bladder, and suprapubic drainage
31. colostomy and partial cystectomy
32. bladder drainage and parenteral hyperalimentation
33. proximal colostomy alone
34. sigmoid resection, proximal colostomy, and bladder drainage
35. transurethral prostatectomy, proximal colostomy, and hyperalimentation

Patient O

A 70-year-old man presented with a history of weakness, fatigue, dark stools, and increasing constipation of 3-months' duration. He has had a long history of constipation, but it has gotten worse recently. He has also had episodes of diarrhea. He had an abdominal operation on a "big blood vessel" 4 years previously; he had a number of x-rays taken at that time and was told that his bowels were "okay for his age." Recently he feels tired all the time and cannot do the things he was able to do previously. He has lost 10 pounds and has been taking vitamins and mineral supplements.

O-1. Additional history of value in diagnosis includes

1. details of previous operation
2. results of bowel x-rays
3. family history
4. nature of bowel movements
5. laxative usage
6. medicines he is taking

O-2. Clinical evaluation should include

7. abdominal distention
8. abdominal mass
9. hepatomegaly
10. ascites
11. rectal examination
12. stool guaiac

O-3. Initial investigations should include (see Figure 3.24)

13. serum electrolytes
14. hemogram
15. serum amylase
16. liver profile
17. chest x-ray
18. plain abdominal series
19. sigmoidoscopy
20. oral cholecystogram (OCG)
21. upper GI series
22. IVP
23. barium enema

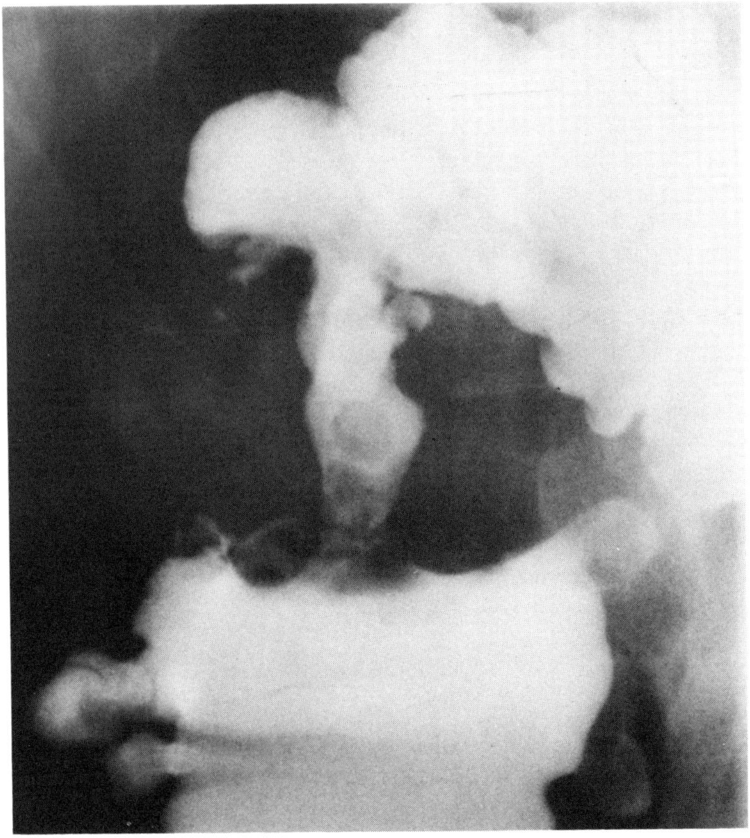

Figure 3.24

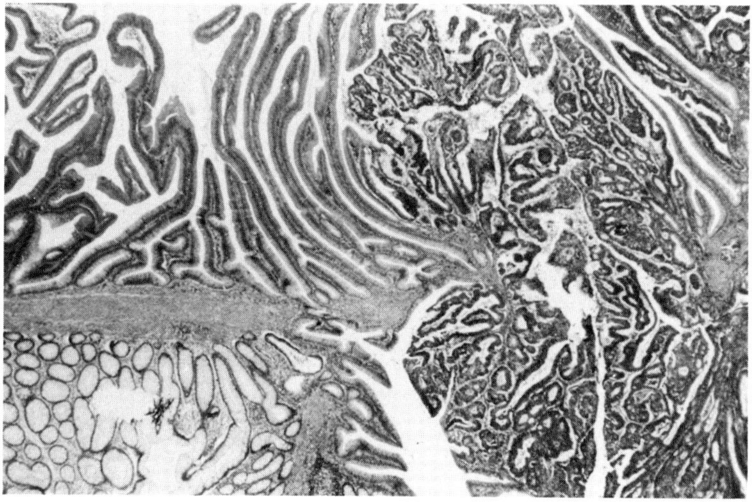

Figure 3.25

O-4. Additional studies and procedures required to confirm the diagnosis are (see Figure 3.25)

24. upper endoscopy and biopsy
25. colonoscopy and biopsy
26. electrolyte replacement
27. serum carcinoembryonic antigen (CEA) levels
28. urinary 5-HIAA levels
29. serum alpha-fetoprotein levels
30. mesenteric angiography
31. transfusion of packed red cells
32. parenteral hyperalimentation
33. mechanical bowel preparation
34. oral antibiotics
35. parenteral vitamin K

O-5. Acceptable methods of treatment include

36. bulk laxatives, antispasmodics, and reevaluation at frequent intervals
37. primary resection and anastomosis
38. abdominoperineal resection
39. first-stage colostomy and drainage, second-stage resection, and third-stage closure of colostomy
40. first-stage resection and colostomy and second-stage closure of colostomy
41. local excision
42. fulguration

O-6. Useful procedures in the follow-up care of this patient include

43. sigmoidoscopy quarterly
44. colonoscopy annually
45. barium enema periodically
46. chest x-ray
47. serum alpha-fetoprotein levels
48. urinary 5-HIAA levels
49. serum CEA levels
50. CT scan quarterly

Scoring System

The scoring system for the patient management problems is designed to reward correct selections and to penalize incorrect selections. Incorrect selections due to omission and commission are both subject to penalty. That is, selecting incorrect actions and not selecting correct actions are both penalized. Selecting or not selecting actions that are optional does not affect the score.

For each correct selection the reader receives one point, and for each incorrect selection loses one point. The final score is determined by taking the sum of the total positive points obtained and subtracting the total negative points obtained, then dividing by the total number of positive points possible times 100. This gives the percentage correct (Proficiency Score) in the patient management section.

\+ = 1 positive point (+1)

− = 1 negative point (−1)

0 = optional (no points)

X = total positive points obtained

Y = total negative points obtained

300 = total positive points possible

$$\text{Proficiency Score (\%)} = \frac{X - Y}{300} \times 100$$

Patient A

Scoring

A-1	A-2	A-3	A-4	A-5
1. +	7. +	13. −	19. +	25. −
2. −	8. +	14. −	20. 0	26. −
3. +	9. −	15. +	21. −	27. +
4. +	10. −	16. +	22. −	28. −
5. −	11. −	17. 0	23. −	29. 0
6. +	12. −	18. 0	24. −	30. −

A-6	A-7	A-8	A-9	A-10
31. +	37. +	44. +	50. −	56. +
32. −	38. −	45. −	51. −	57. +
33. +	39. −	46. −	52. −	58. +
34. −	40. +	47. −	53. −	59. +
35. −	41. 0	48. −	54. −	60. +
36. −	42. +	49. 0	55. +	61. +
	43. +			

Discussion

This case illustrates the value of combining radiography, echocardiography, fluoroscopy, and cineangiography to document findings consistent with that of prosthetic valvular dehiscence, confirmed at surgery.

Strict attention to detail and frequent serial examinations of the patient are imperative in the evaluation of prosthetic valve function. Only with repeated evaluations will changes in auscultation, x-rays, echocardiograms, and other noninvasive examinations be evident. Valvular dysfunction varies from obstruction to gross valvular dehiscence, as in this patient. Familiarity with the prosthesis facilitates an expeditious diagnosis of the malfunction. Of interest is the dramatic deterioration of the patient despite the presence of normal prosthetic sounds and the absence of a murmur.

The x-ray revealed the patient to be in florid pulmonary edema and to have an exaggerated tilting of his valve (see Figure 3.2). The echocardiogram revealed a characteristic "hump" on the prosthetic valve echo consistent with frank dehiscence of the prosthesis (see Figure 3.3). Cinefluoroscopy was invaluable in detecting excessive cyclic excursion of the sewing ring (see Figures 3.4 and 3.5).

The detachment of the valve prosthesis was probably brought about by the strain in the sutures in the anchoring tissue resulting from the force of ventricular contraction. In the mitral position, the strain on the suture line is greatest at the medial and lateral aspects of the sewing ring. If the suture breaks in one of these locations, as in this patient, it puts a strain on the adjacent sutures, causing progressive dehiscence and possibly leading to complete detachment and embolization of the entire prosthesis.

Although contrast angiography is the most sensitive indicator of prosthetic valvular detachment, radiography, echocardiography, fluoroscopy, and cineangiography should be used in all suspected cases. Serial studies with the foregoing noninvasive procedures, beginning with an early postoperative control study, are recommended.

Patient B

Scoring

B-1	B-2	B-3	B-4	B-5	B-6
1. 0	7. +	14. 0	21. 0	28. −	34. −
2. +	8. +	15. 0	22. 0	29. 0	35. +
3. +	9. 0	16. −	23. −	30. 0	36. −
4. +	10. +	17. −	24. 0	31. −	37. +
5. −	11. +	18. 0	25. −	32. +	38. +
6. +	12. +	19. 0	26. −	33. −	39. +
	13. +	20. 0	27. +		40. +

Discussion

Psoriasis can easily be worsened by improper management. Systemic corticosteroids are beneficial immediately but usually cause a rebound when withdrawn. The lesions also usually flare with trauma, so gentle cleansing is sufficient. Most psoriasis can be controlled with tar shampoos, bath oils, and topical corticosteroids. Skin of the face and genitalia may atrophy from prolonged use of potent topical steroids. Consequently, only milder formulations, such as 1% hydrocortisone, should be used on lesions in these locations. Stronger steroids are needed to heal the thicker plaques usually found on the trunk, elbows, knees, and sometimes scalp.

Cases that fail to respond to topical treatment may require intralesional steroids, ultraviolet light therapy, retinoids, and even methotrexate. These treatments, with their numerous potential side effects, are best administered by a dermatologist.

Patient C

Scoring

C-1	C-2	C-3	C-4	C-5	C-6
1. +	7. +	13. +	20. +	25. 0	29. +
2. +	8. +	14. +	21. −	26. +	30. +
3. +	9. +	15. +	22. +	27. +	31. −
4. 0	10. +	16. 0	23. −	28. −	32. 0
5. +	11. 0	17. 0	24. 0		
6. −	12. −	18. −			
		19. +			

Discussion

This woman presents with a history of acute onset of arthritis. All sorts of etiologic possibilities come to mind, such as rheumatic, rheumatoid, infectious, and traumatic. The history of coincidental hives points toward a serum sickness reaction but does not in any way pinpoint the etiology. The absence of any history of drugs or medication is no help. The physical exam confirms that there is not only arthralgia, but also real arthritis with effusion evident in her knee. The need to rule out some collagen disease is apparent and even an infectious etiology, such as gonococcal arthritis, is not excluded. It is the screening laboratory work which puts things into perspective. The elevation of the SGOT and bilirubin points toward underlying infective (viral) hepatitis. This is strengthened as an explanation for her arthritis by the relative lymphocytosis and the negative latex and ANA.

A serum sicknesslike syndrome is a frequent prodromal presentation of viral hepatitis. Various studies give an incidence ranging from 10% to 20%, and these are probably conservative estimates if one considers the frequency of inapparent hepatitis that goes undiagnosed. Quick confirmation is obtained with the positive HBsAg. The diagnosis is acute viral hepatitis type B. Neither the positive anti-HBc or negative anti-HBe is of great clinical significance at this time because this pattern of reactivity is expected with acute disease. Antibody against core antigen is an early response and may be present in low titer before symptoms appear. It will persist in individuals with chronic infection. Early in the infection this antibody is an IgM, while in chronic disease it is usually an IgG. Assays for anti-HBc IgM are available and can be of use in separating acute from chronic infection in patients that present with an incidental finding of a positive HBsAg. The utility of assays for e antigen and anti-HBe rests with the conversion from the presence of HBeAg to anti-HBeAg. This conversion marks the beginning of recovery and the onset of remission of the hepatitis infection. In this patient, it is too early to expect anti-e to be present.

Liver biopsy is unnecessary. The diagnosis has been made by demonstrating the infective virus, and even though the risks of liver biopsy are very small, they are unjustified in this case at this time.

The cornerstone of management of a patient with viral hepatitis remains rest, adequate nutrition, and careful follow-up. Regimens of strict enforced bed rest have given way to a much more reasoned balance of restricted activity and self-care. Each case does need to be individualized to its social setting as well as to the clinical severity of the hepatitis. Rapid progressive deterioration warrants hospitalization, but the overwhelming percentage of patients can be treated at home. In this case, the assistance of a cooperative roommate and a solicitous boyfriend permitted treatment at home.

Hepatitis is a slow-moving process. Early in the process, evaluation at weekly intervals avoids the surprise of rapid progression. As the infection stabilizes and, particularly, begins to wane, reevaluation need be less frequent. Patients should be followed until liver function returns to normal. In addition to enzymes and bilirubin, serial prothrombin times can be sensitive indicators of deterioration of liver function.

Two epidemiologic features need to be considered. First, has this infection come from a point source that might involve others? While this was not included in the discussion, no point source was identified. Second, what should be said to patient contacts, or really, should prophylaxis be offered? Important points need to be considered. First, type A hepatitis remains a common enough experience that pooled gamma globulin is useful in prophylaxis and is relatively inexpensive for this purpose. Pooled gamma globulin is not useful in the prophylaxis of hepatitis B. Preparations of hyperimmune globulin are required. These are expensive. Second, while type B is directly transmissable person to person, it does require intimacy. Virus is present in saliva, blood, and semen. Accordingly, the boyfriend is at greatest risk and should be offered prophylaxis. The patient's roommate may be at slightly smaller risk; however, sharing food preparation and eating utensils, and toilet and bathing facilities with the patient would prompt an offer of prophylaxis. This is a judgment call and some physicians might not think the risk significant. Casual contacts, fellow classmates, and students are not considered at risk.

As the story unfolds, her hepatitis has taken on a chronic character. Her activity remains restricted by the need to return to bed rest with each clinical flare of activity. She has had several visits to a gastroenterologist, and now at 6 months she has had a biopsy that is compatible with chronic active hepatitis. The choice of starting steroids now or waiting another 3 to 6 months, then performing another biopsy, is not easy. Some bouts of hepatitis B do take 6 months or more to resolve, yet the "bridging" present on the biopsy is a bad sign. The prospect of high-dose steroids for years is not without its dangers. A conservative approach would include waiting at least another 3 months and perform another biopsy before deciding.

Patient D

Scoring

D-1	D-2	D-3	D-4	D-5	D-6
1. 0	5. +	11. +	19. −	25. +	30. +
2. −	6. −	12. +	20. −	26. −	31. 0
3. −	7. −	13. +	21. −	27. −	32. −
4. −	8. +	14. +	22. −	28. +	33. +
	9. −	15. −	23. 0	29. −	34. +
	10. +	16. +	24. 0		35. −
		17. +			
		18. −			

D-7	D-8	D-9	D-10	D-11	D-12
36. 0	41. +	44. −	61. −	63. −	71. −
37. 0	42. −	45. +	62. −	64. +	72. −
38. 0	43. +	46. +		65. +	73. +
39. 0		47. +		66. −	74. −
40. +		48. +		67. +	75. 0
		49. +		68. −	76. +
		50. +		69. −	77. −
		51. +		70. +	78. +
		52. 0			
		53. −			
		54. +			
		55. −			
		56. 0			
		57. −			
		58. −			
		59. −			
		60. −			

Discussion

The initial assessment of this patient begins with the information obtained from this history and physical examination. She is a known diabetic of many years duration who presents with symptoms of urinary tract disease. The length of her history of diabetes itself would make you think of the possibility of renal disease, and this would most likely be diabetic glomerulosclerosis (with a probability of more than 90%). Her symptoms, however, suggest not this diagnosis but a lower urinary tract disease, and with her fever, this is most likely an infection.

The most important diagnostic test at this time, then, is the collection of a clean-catch urine and a simple urinalysis looking for WBC. If a stain such as Sternheimer-Malbin is available, the presence of "glitter" cells can be determined, but the mere presence of WBC should be enough to make a tentative diagnosis. If bacteria are seen, then the diagnosis is even more certain, and you would then also know that the colony count was probably 100,000/mL or more.

In addition, if oval fat bodies or "maltese crosses" were seen, a further confirmation of diabetic glomerulosclerosis could be made. A 24-hour urinary protein excretion would help in establishing a diagnosis of diabetic nephropathy, if the protein content were greater than 3 g/24 hr.

Further work-up now consists of determining how to manage the patient because the diagnosis can be made with the urinalysis. A urine culture is necessary to determine the organism(s) present and the antibiotic sensitivity of each. Meanwhile, because the patient is symptomatic and febrile, an antibiotic can be started. The choice now is whether to start only one or several drugs. The chances are that if she has not been instrumented a single drug will be enough. Since the most common organism in urinary tract infections is *Escherichia coli*, ampicillin would be a good choice if she is not allergic to the penicillin group of antibiotics. This then could be started to await the results of the cultures. Other treatments, such as antipyretics or analgesics, could be used to alleviate symptoms. If the organism is sensitive to the antibiotic, the temperature should fall in about 24 hours. Otherwise, with the culture results, which should be available within 24 to 48 hours, another antibiotic can be added or substituted.

After the initial problem is taken care of, the assessment of her renal function can be done. Again, simple tests should be done first. A serum creatinine would tell you whether she has much renal failure. A serum creatinine greater than 1.0 mg/dL would make you suspicious of renal impairment and a creatinine clearance would be indicated. If the serum creatinine were greater than 3.0 mg/dL, a decreased creatinine clearance would be expected and a rough estimate of clearance could be made by the following empirical calculation:

$$\text{Clearance} = (140 - \text{age}) \times \text{wt(kg)}/\text{serum creatinine} \times 72$$

A creatinine clearance would be essential if the serum creatinine were between 1.0 and 3.0 because between these points the relation of clearance and serum creatinine is unreliable.

A renal biopsy could be done but is not necessary. If in doubt, a biopsy would confirm the diagnosis of diabetic glomerulosclerosis, which is what the photomicrograph shows. In the presence of findings that do not fit the usual picture of diabetic glomerulosclerosis, a biopsy may be indicated to rule out a treatable disease. In one series, this is possible in about 4% of instances. In this same series, about 8% had another disease together with diabetic glomerulosclerosis.

The patient was started on an antibiotic (ampicillin) and responded with a drop in temperature and a clearing of her urine of bacteria and WBC. A repeat urine culture would be helpful but not absolutely necessary at this time to determine if her urine was now sterile.

However, she now develops a complication and returns with diarrhea, most likely due to the antibiotic. This has resulted in a sufficient loss of fluid that she has postural hypotension and poor skin turgor, suggesting that she has lost 10% or more of her body weight in water. A very rough estimate of water loss is that thirst and dry mouth occur at a loss of about 5% of body weight or less, and signs such as poor skin turgor occur at a loss of 10% or more. Postural hypotension most likely represents a greater loss. Knowing her previous weight and obtaining her present weight would give an estimate of her water loss (remembering that she had had 2+ edema and that she was placed on a diuretic during her last admission).

Her problem at this time is more likely to be one of water and electrolyte imbalance. For this reason, you should determine her serum sodium, chloride, and bicarbonate. A serum potassium and serum osmolality would also be helpful, but none of the other electrolytes will provide much more useful information. If her serum sodium is elevated, dehydration is a good bet.

With the current weight and her serum sodium (if elevated), a rough estimate of her water deficit can be calculated. If her serum sodium is high, as one would expect with water loss, then the following formula will give an estimate of her water loss:

$$V = [wt(kg) \times 0.6] - [wt(kg) \times 0.6 \times Na^+]/140$$

where V $=$ volume deficit
wt $=$ weight in kilograms
Na^+ $=$ measured sodium
0.6 $=$ total body water (60%)

If the result from this calculation is similar to the previous gross estimates, then initially any sodium loss can be ignored and rehydration started slowly with about ½ of the value derived from the formula in the first 24 hours. If the serum sodium is not high and especially if she has a low bicarbonate (due to GI loss of HCO_3^-), then the formula will not give an accurate estimate and she will need water, sodium, and bicarbonate. Under these circumstances it would be best to begin to correct her sodium/bicarbonate deficit by giving half normal saline plus sodium bicarbonate to make it isotonic or 5% dextrose in water plus sodium bicarbonate. After 12 and 24 hours a repeat determination of her serum sodium and bicarbonate would give another set of values from which the same formula would again give an estimate of her water loss as well as her sodium and bicarbonate status. At this point again the same reasoning could be used and either bicarbonate or water given in about ½ the estimated amount.

Rehydration should be done slowly to avoid cerebral edema as a result of the presence of idiogenic osmols in the brain parenchyma. Correction of her bicarbonate loss acidosis most likely could be accomplished first by parenteral means but later by oral bicarbonate. Whenever feasible it is better to correct such abnormalities by oral means.

Since the information provided shows a decrease in bicarbonate, a blood pH and pCO_2 would be helpful. The results of these studies show a non-anion gap acidosis with a high serum chloride. The most likely cause for this bicarbonate loss is her diarrhea, very likely due to the antibiotic that she was taking.

Treatment consists of stopping the diarrhea and replacing the bicarbonate. The antibiotic should be stopped and an antidiarrheal agent added if necessary. Oral sodium bicarbonate can be given or, if necessary, sodium bicarbonate could be given IV.

One method of calculating the dose of bicarbonate is

$$\text{Dose } NaHCO_3 = HCO_3^- = \frac{\text{deficit} \times \text{wt} \times 0.5}{2}.$$

This is given over several hours, and the determination and calculations are repeated.

A number of answers have been considered as either not helpful or as unnecessary. In general, this is based on the premise that only information that is directly associated with making a diagnosis or instituting therapy is correct. With this in mind, the following were considered in this category: 1–4, 6, 7, 9, 15, 18–22, 32, 36–39, 42, 44, 53, 55, 58–62, 71, 72.

Several answers are wrong: 26, 27, 29, 63, 65, 68, 69.

Answer 66 could be considered, at least from the standpoint of the presence of a non-anion gap hyperchloremic acidosis, to possibly represent renal tubular acidosis. This would have to exist in the presence of diabetic glomerulosclerosis and an elevated serum creatinine and would therefore be a type 4 renal tubular acidosis. Other findings would not support this diagnosis.

References

1. Stamm WE, Turck M: Urinary tract infection, pyelonephritis, and related conditions, in Braunwald E, et al. (eds): *Harrison's Principles of Internal Medicine*, ed 11. New York, McGraw-Hill, 1987, pp 1189–1195.

2. Kasinath BS, et al: Nondiabetic renal disease in patients with diabetes mellitus. *Am J Med* 1983;75:613–617.

3. Antonovych TT, Mostofi FK: *Atlas of Kidney Biopsies*. Washington, DC, Armed Forces Institute of Pathology, 1980, pp 297–306.

4. Kern TS, Engerman RL: Kidney morphology in experimental hypertension. *Diabetes* 1987;36:244–249.

5. Hruska K: Pathology of acid-base metabolism, in Klahr S (ed): *The Kidney and Body Fluids*. New York, Plenum, 1983, pp 223–267.

6. Morgensen CE, Christensen CK: Predicting diabetic nephropathy in insulin-dependent patients. *N Engl J Med* 1984; 311:89–93.

7. Spooner RJ, Weir RJ, Frier BM: Detection of microalbuminuria in diabetic patients using a simple latex agglutination test. *Clin Chim Acta* 1987;166:247–253.

Patient E

Scoring

E-1	E-2	E-3	E-4	E-5
1. 0	6. +	13. 0	21. 0	34. 0
2. 0	7. −	14. +	22. 0	35. −
3. +	8. 0	15. 0	23. 0	36. −
4. −	9. 0	16. +	24. +	37. +
5. 0	10. +	17. +	25. +	38. 0
	11. +	18. +	26. +	39. 0
	12. 0	19. +	27. +	
		20. +	28. +	
			29. +	
			30. 0	
			31. +	
			32. +	
			33. 0	

E-6	E-7	E-8	E-9	E-10
40. +	47. −	56. −	62. −	67. −
41. +	48. +	57. −	63. −	68. 0
42. 0	49. +	58. −	64. +	69. +
43. 0	50. −	59. +	65. −	70. 0
44. −	51. −	60. −	66. −	
45. +	52. −	61. −		
46. +	53. +			
	54. +			
	55. +			

Discussion

The early symptoms of this patient are typical of giant cell (cranial) arteritis: muscle stiffness, soreness, weight loss, malaise, anorexia, and fleeting head and other pains. Early diagnosis is essential because of the possibility of sudden and devastating visual loss, which can occur at any time. The eye pains of recent onset here suggest that such an emergency is brewing. Thus, the only reason to interrupt the flow of history-taking is to draw a blood sample for ESR because almost always this is greatly increased. None of the responses in E-2 are of particular value except 10; you will have to be very careful giving steroids to a patient with a history of peptic ulcer symptoms. This condition is called giant cell arteritis because not only the cranial arteries and certainly not only the temporal arteries are affected, but also the coronary, renal, and any peripheral vessels may be involved (see Figure 3.26). The neck symptoms and nocturia in E-3 are incidental, as is

Figure 3.26. (Patient E) Cranial arteritis. Biopsy of superficial temporal artery. The lumen is greatly narrowed and the wall is infiltrated by inflammatory cells, including prominent multinucleated giant cells. Paraffin section is stained with hematoxylin and eosin ×65. Inset: giant cell, histiocytes, and lymphocytes ×165. (Courtesy of Dr. Gordon Mathieson.)

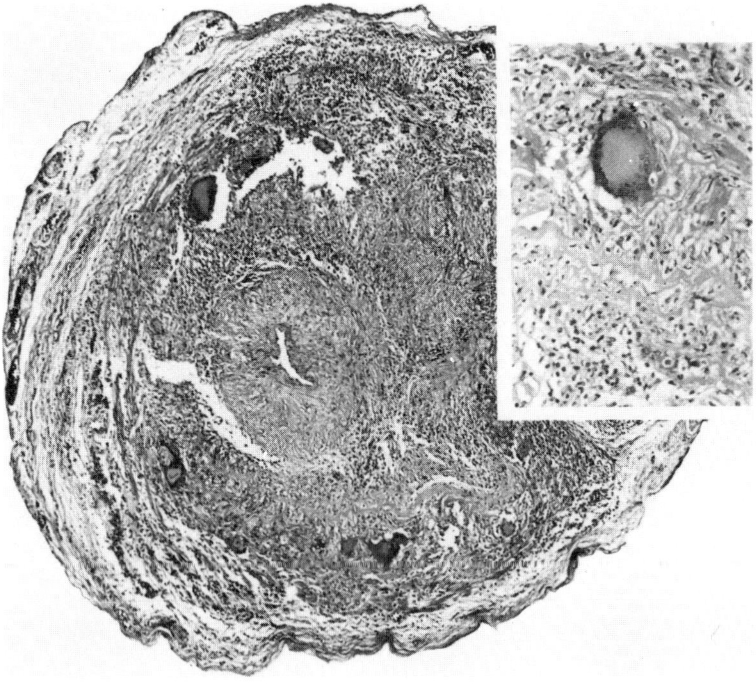

the asymptomatic carotid bruit in E-4 but 24 to 28 all relate to possible findings.

You doubtless want to relieve the man's headache after examining him, but the signs so far should have made you alert to the correct diagnosis and you would be entirely justified in giving high-dose steroids even before the ESR result returns and certainly before the temporal artery biopsy results are at hand. This is likely to prevent visual loss and will relieve pain better than anything else.

Among all the investigations, the ESR and muscle biopsy or arterial biopsy are the only ones of diagnostic importance. Asymptomatic bruits have not been shown to be better treated by surgery, so no angiography is necessary. Likewise, CT scanning is not necessary; it is rather a luxury, though an isotope flow study may be of interest and will at least practically rule out any supratentorial mass lesion.

Adult-onset migraine probably causes at least as much in the way of neurologic deficit as it causes head pain and is a difficult diagnosis best made by exclusion. The elevation in BP here is not nearly enough to cause severe headaches; nor would cervical spondylosis be blamed for persistent headaches until all other likely causes have been excluded. A mass lesion is unlikely with a normal CNS examination and with venous pulses present, more or less excluding significantly raised intracranial pressure. Hydrocephalus ex vacuo does not cause headache.

The only therapy is steroids, in high dosage initially. Polymyalgia rheumatica, a variant of this syndrome, may improve on low doses, but the risk to sight remains until all arteritis is suppressed; to achieve this, you must give initially 80 mg to 100 mg of prednisolone daily, tapering the dose after months so long as the ESR is reduced to normal values and the clinical symptoms are suppressed. An H_2 receptor antagonist should also be given. That done, the long-term prognosis is good and the disease may be expected to burn itself out within 3 to 5 years in most cases.

Patient F

Scoring

F-1	F-2	F-3	F-4	F-5	F-6
1. +	9. +	16. −	22. +	27. −	32. −
2. +	10. +	17. +	23. −	28. 0	33. −
3. 0	11. +	18. 0	24. −	29. +	34. +
4. 0	12. −	19. +	25. −	30. −	35. 0
5. 0	13. +	20. −	26. −	31. −	36. −
6. +	14. −	21. +			37. 0
7. +	15. +				
8. −					

Discussion

Third trimester bleeding is often a very difficult and perplexing problem for the physician. On the one hand, you wish to stop the bleeding; while on the other, you must worry about fetal maturity and survival.

When a patient presents with third trimester bleeding, it is essential that noninvasive procedures be utilized to make the diagnosis. In a multiparous patient, the most likely cause is placenta previa. However, premature separation can also occur in multiparous patients and previa in primigravidas. Other causes of bleeding are usually uncommon or rare. As a result, most diagnostic tests should be directed toward these two entities.

Since ultrasound has such a high degree of accuracy, it should be your first procedure. Although in the past, amniograms and double setups played an important role, they should no longer be considered. Once the diagnosis is made, then a definitive course of treatment can be undertaken.

Patient G

Scoring

G-1	G-2	G-3	G-4	G-5	G-6
1. +	7. +	13. +	19. +	25. –	31. –
2. +	8. 0	14. –	20. +	26. +	32. –
3. 0	9. –	15. 0	21. –	27. –	33. –
4. +	10. 0	16. –	22. –	28. –	34. +
5. +	11. 0	17. +	23. –	29. –	35. 0
6. –	12. 0	18. 0	24. +	30. –	36. –

Discussion

Sudden acute abdominal pain in a young woman should always be suspected of being associated with an ectopic tubal pregnancy until proven otherwise. A similar symptom can occur with pelvic infection, torsion of an ovarian cyst, renal colic, appendicitis, and other abdominal problems. However, none of these is imminently life threatening and the patient can undergo an evaluation. With an ectopic pregnancy, the outcome can be rapidly fatal. As a result, all of the initial evaluation should be aimed at diagnosing whether or not this is an ectopic gestation. In many series this will result in a misdiagnosis in up to one fourth of cases. However, this should not be considered a determinant of procedures but a necessary part of the prevention. It is far better to make the diagnosis in error than it is to miss the diagnosis.

Although ectopic pregnancy means a pregnancy in any site other than the uterine cavity, it is usually a tubal implantation (98%) and thus used synonymously with tubal pregnancy. The etiology of the disease is usually a disease or procedure that alters ovum transport and predisposes to a tubal implantation. The most common causes are pelvic infection and tubal surgery. The incidence of the disease varies depending on the patient population and ranges from 1 in 40 to 1 in 300 deliveries. The incidence appears to be increasing; this is thought to be due to the increasing incidence of pelvic infections from sexually transmitted diseases and intrauterine devices, as well as the greater frequency of tubal surgery.

Diagnosis of the disease may be confusing because the symptoms are common to many other diseases. The most common symptom is abdominal pain (95%). Other symptoms include a pelvic mass (50%), abdominal bleeding (75%), and delayed menses (60%). Additional complaints include shoulder pain (25%), nausea (20%), and syncope (10%). None of this by itself or in association with others is diagnostic. The classic triad of amenorrhea, bleeding, and abdominal pain should always lead the physician to suspect ectopic pregnancy until proven otherwise.

Laboratory tests should include a hemoglobin and hematocrit, which may be less than normal due to intraperitoneal bleeding, and a qualitative beta HCG. Urine pregnancy tests are helpful if positive but are usually negative at this stage of pregnancy and so can be misleading.

Whenever an ectopic pregnancy is suspected, an ultrasound should be performed. This test can detect an intrauterine pregnancy and help make the diagnosis. It can also indicate a tubal pregnancy, but this is not as accurate as intrauterine detection. Another very useful procedure is a culdocentesis. The presence of nonclotting blood is diagnostic of an intraperitoneal hemorrhage and requires immediate intervention. A paracentesis can also be used but is far less helpful because small quantities of blood in the pelvis are easily missed.

If the diagnosis is still in doubt, then a diagnostic laparoscopy should be performed. A good rule to follow with a suspected ectopic pregnancy is when in doubt—laparoscopy.

Treatment of an ectopic pregnancy is excision and removal. If bleeding is profuse, a transfusion is also indicated. Currently there is debate about when to remove the pregnancy and leave the tube and when to remove the tube with the pregnancy. There are many arguments on both sides, but most physicians will always remove the tube if it has begun to rupture and only leave an early unruptured tube. In the past, the ovary was always removed and, with a repeat ectopic pregnancy, a hysterectomy was performed. Recent advances with in vitro fertilization have changed this view, and the ovaries and uterus should be left.

Patient H

Scoring

H-1	H-2	H-3	H-4	H-5	H-6
1. 0	8. +	14. −	20. 0	28. −	34. −
2. +	9. −	15. −	21. 0	29. +	35. +
3. +	10. +	16. +	22, +	30. −	36. +
4. 0	11. 0	17. +	23. +	31. −	37. +
5. 0	12. −	18. −	24. 0	32. −	38. −
6. 0	13. −	19. 0	25. −	33. 0	39. −
7. 0			26. +		
			27. +		

Discussion

Pregnancy-induced hypertension (PIH) is still one of the most complex problems facing the physician today. Since the etiology is unknown, the treatment and management remain empirical. This disease was originally referred to as preeclampsia or toxemia, and eclampsia if a convulsion occurred. We now know that there is no toxin in the blood, so toxemia is incorrect. Since the underlying cause may be multiple and may occur with preexisting diseases, the term pregnancy-induced hypertension makes a much more accurate nomenclature. Eclampsia is still used once a convulsion takes place.

The major diagnostic criterion is an elevation in blood pressure. This must be present on more than one occasion and at least 6 hours apart (some authors now state only 1 hour). Hypertension is present when the systolic pressure reads 140 mmHg or increases by 30 mmHg, and/or the diastolic pressure reaches 90 mmHg or increases by 15 mmHg. These changes are considered mild until the blood pressure reaches 160/110, then it is considered severe. The presence of edema either on examination or as evidenced by sudden weight gain is also part of the disease but not necessary to make the diagnosis. Proteinuria of 30 mg/L in a 24-hour urine specimen is also part of the triad but not essential to the diagnosis.

PIH of some degree occurs in 1% to 10% of all deliveries, depending on the type of patients studied. There is a higher incidence in primigravidas, in women less than 18 and over 35 years of age, in multiple pregnancies, with preexisting vascular diseases, with hydatidiform mole, and in hydraminos.

The disease is manifested as primarily a change in blood pressure, but other organ systems are also involved. The kidneys develop glomerular changes; liver damage may be severe; cerebral changes, including visual disturbances and edema, can occur; the coagulating system may be altered; and premature placental separation is common.

The usual clinical course of the disease is a progressive elevation in blood pressure, especially the diastolic. This may be associated with edema and sudden weight gain, as well as proteinuria. As the disease progresses, and it may do so rapidly, the patient may notice oliguria, headache, visual disturbances such as flashing yellow and green lights, and abdominal pain (liver capsule distention). These secondary signs are often the herald of an impending convulsion.

The most significant laboratory findings are related to the effect on the kidneys. Proteinemia will increase kidney function tests, such as the BUN; creatinine and uric acid become elevated; and the hematocrit and platelets may also be altered. Coagulant defects may also occur, but these are usually the end result of premature separation of the placenta rather than of the disease itself.

The differential diagnosis is not difficult because most patients are healthy young adults without previous problems. Conditions to be considered include chronic hypertensive vascular disease, nephrosis, glomerulonephritis, lupus, and pheochromocytoma.

Treatment of the disease should first be aimed at prevention. This includes adequate rest, diet, and frequent monitoring. Once the disease occurs, then treatment can be divided into two phases: home and hospital. Treatment consists of bed rest and salt reduction (not elimination). It has a limited role and is only used for those patients who are in the earliest of stages where the diagnosis is not established. These patients must be seen frequently (at least every 2 to 3 days) and any worsening requires hospitalization immediately.

Hospital care is necessary for all cases of overt PIH. Treatment must be designed to reduce the hypertension, correct the physiologic balance, reduce the instability, and prevent the complications, especially convulsion. To accomplish all of these, the patient needs intensive care in the labor and delivery suite, not on a general nursing floor. She should be placed at bed rest in the lateral recumbent position with continuous fetal monitoring. Fluid intake, urinary output, and reflexes should be measured and recorded. The initial drugs of choice should include IV magnesium sulfate, hydralazine, and a diuretic. Diet should be high protein with sodium restriction to less than 0.5–1 g/d.

The ultimate treatment is delivery. The exact timing will depend on the severity of the disease, the ability to stabilize the patient, and the improvement. The method of choice is usually elective induction; however, many patients will ultimately have a cesarean section.

Patient I

Scoring

I-1	I-2	I-3	I-4	I-5	I-6
1. +	9. +	17. 0	24. +	31. −	35. −
2. +	10. +	18. +	25. +	32. +	36. −
3. +	11. +	19. −	26. −	33. −	37. +
4. 0	12. +	20. −	27. −	34. 0	38. +
5. 0	13. −	21. −	28. −		39. 0
6. −	14. +	22. +	29. −		
7. 0	15. +	23. +	30. +		
8. +	16. +				

Discussion

The case presented is that of an adolescent girl who is involved in a car accident and who is brought to the emergency room for attention. Her vital signs are quite stable, and there is thus no need for immediate emergency management. History taking at this time needs to be directed to circumstances of the accident, especially any loss of consciousness, in order to assess the situation adequately. It is always appropriate to put pediatric patients in perspective by inquiring about allergies, past hospitalizations, family history, and a brief review of systems. The few minutes that these questions take often pay off in terms of a more thorough assessment of the patient. Before establishing a relationship with an adolescent, it is not appropriate to suggest abuse of drugs unless emergency management dictates it. In this case, the history reveals that the patient has had some vague abdominal discomfort for a few months.

On physical exam, we learn that there is some pinpoint rib tenderness, a few abrasions on the head and extremities, and some vague abdominal pain. The rectal exam is probably not indicated at this point in dealing with the case because there is no absolute medical reason to perform it and this is better done at a later point when more of a relationship has been established. The laboratory studies should reflect what has been learned from the history and physical. There does not appear to be any injury suggestive of excessive blood loss, but one could not argue with the desire for a

CBC as a baseline. A skull x-ray is not indicated in view of the history (no loss of consciousness) and physical exam. The chest x-ray, although negative, is indicated in view of the trauma and pain expressed on physical exam. Abdominal films at this time are unlikely to be helpful; the findings are vague and not at all suggestive of serious intraabdominal pathology (such as a ruptured spleen). In addition, the patient has complained of vague pain for a few months. An ECG is not indicated because the murmur described is typical of a functional murmur, which is a common finding in adolescence. Urinalysis is simple, easy, inexpensive, and can be revealing whenever there is any suggestion of renal trauma. Culture of the vaginal discharge is indicated, even though it is not part of the original complaint.

As the case progresses, it is important to retake the vital signs, especially in view of the slight elevation in blood pressure originally found. The immunization history, which was not asked initially, needs to be obtained in order to assess the need for tetanus toxoid. Psychiatric consult and typing for blood have no place in the management of this case; she has acted quite reasonably, and there is nothing to suggest serious blood loss. Cardiology and neurologic consults are also unnecessary at this point; there have been essentially normal findings in these areas. In view of the vaginal discharge, it is very important that additional sexual history be obtained in a straightforward, confidential, gentle manner. This is one of the important keys in proper management of this case. Adolescents may enter the health care system in a variety of ways, and one must always entertain the possibility that an adolescent girl presenting with a totally different complaint may indeed be pregnant. There are approximately 1 million pregnancies each year among adolescents, with over 10% in young women under 15 years of age. The fact that this girl is a Tanner stage 5 (Table 3.2) and has a vaginal discharge demands further investigation.

Further management thus leads to a pregnancy test. IVP and a CT scan are not indicated because the extent of injuries is limited. If one felt uncertain about the abdominal findings one could satisfy oneself with a surgical opinion. It is quite possible to miss a pregnancy on a physical exam in the first trimester, especially if one is not looking for it; rectal and vaginal exams are not routinely performed on every adolescent girl unless a relationship has been established or there is a definite indication from the history or circumstances. The rectal exam in this girl revealed hard stools,

TABLE 3.2. Tanner Sex Maturity Stages in Girls

Stage	Pubic hair	Breasts
1	Preadolescent	Preadolescent
2	Sparse, lightly pigmented, straight	Breast elevated as a small mound, areolar diameter increased
3	Darker, increased amount, beginning to curl	Breast and areolar enlarged, no separation of contours
4	Coarse, curly, abundant	Areolar and papilla form secondary mound
5	Adult female triangle, spread to medial surface of thighs	Mature: nipple projects, areolar part of breast contours

and the enlarged uterus was not appreciated. Vaginal exam was not done, and the uterus was not yet big enough to be felt on abdominal exam.

Proper management includes dressing the wounds and counseling about head trauma because even trauma such as that described can result in delayed onset of symptoms. Admission or further observation in the emergency room with an IV running are not indicated in view of the benign course of the injuries. It is essential that the adolescent be referred for proper counseling. At this point, it is important to maintain the patient's confidentiality. She should be encouraged to share the diagnosis of pregnancy with her parents, but if she does not want to, that decision should be respected. Informing the social worker of the situation will help ensure follow-up.

In summary, whenever dealing with an adolescent for a medical problem, a good sexual history must be gently obtained in an open, confidential manner in order to provide proper medical assessment and care. In the case presented, a girl brought to the emergency room because of trauma turned out to have minimal injuries but was pregnant, alone, and in need of help and counseling.

Patient J

Scoring

J-1	J-2	J-3	J-4	J-5	J-6
1. 0	13. +	21. −	34. −	40. −	48. +
2. +	14. −	22. −	35. −	41. +	49. +
3. +	15. −	23. 0	36. −	42. −	50. +
4. 0	16. −	24. −	37. 0	43. +	51. +
5. −	17. 0	25. 0	38. +	44. 0	52. −
6. +	18. +	26. −	39. −	45. +	53. −
7. 0	19. +	27. −		46. +	54. 0
8. +	20. +	28. +		47. +	55. +
9. +		29. +			56. +
10. +		30. 0			57. −
11. +		31. +			58. +
12. +		32. +			
		33. +			

Discussion

The case presented is that of a sexually active teenage boy who comes for treatment of a sexually transmitted disease (STD). As always, taking a good history is critical to treating the patient appropriately. Reviewing his immunization status is not so important to his present illness, but it is part of practicing good medicine. There have been a number of outbreaks of measles recently on college campuses, because of young people who were born after 1956 (and therefore are presumed to not have natural immunity) and who did not receive the vaccine. Review of allergy history is especially important, since penicillin may be a drug given to treat an STD. General review of systems is always helpful to be sure that there are no areas worthy of further evaluation. His record of past hospitalizations again is useful to place his overall medical condition in context.

Many people feel that any contact with an adolescent demands a special history, abbreviated HEADS (home, education & employment, activities, drugs, and sexuality). A quick review of these areas with appropriate questioning will give a good sense of how the young person is coping with adolescence. Question J-5 is scored negatively because of the form the question takes, which allows the teen to answer with one word, accomplishing nothing. "What are you good (bad) at in school?" is a better way to elicit information. The form of the question about substance abuse is better because it is open-ended and specific enough to get information, creating an opportunity to deliver a strong "no drugs" message. Asking about previous urinary tract infections (UTIs) is unlikely to be helpful in this situation. UTI symptoms in a female must always be distinguished from dysuria syndrome caused by chlamydia. Onset of symptoms is always important as is timing of any medication taken, which may affect culture results.

A complete sexual history is very important. It should include starting with the question: "Have you had sexual relations with anyone? Do you have sex with men, women, or both?" This is a nonjudgmental, straightforward way of getting the needed information. One then proceeds to ask about a current steady sexual partner, and how many partners in the last month(s). Next one must identify sites at risk. In our patient, all three sites are at risk. Specific questions are often needed to determine this. "Did you put your penis in his (her) mouth? Did you put your penis in his rectum? Did he put his penis in your mouth? Did he put his penis in your rectum? Were condoms used, and if so did they break?" So a good sexual history determines: (1) if the individual is having sexual relationships; (2) sexual orientation; (3) if there is a current steady partner; (4) number of recent partners; (5) sites at risk; (6) safer sex practices; and one could also include (7) any concerns about sexual dysfunction.

In the physical exam, one would be concerned about a thorough examination of the genitalia and rectum. Pharyngeal gonorrhea (GC) is often unremarkable on exam. Funduscopic exam in this situation is pointless, as is the search for CVA tenderness, and joint mobility (GC arthritis is not subtle). The critical laboratory tests are GC cultures of all sites at risk, and a gram stain of the urethral discharge. Doing a fluorescent type chlamydial test, looking for elementary bodies will depend on cost and availability. It is not essential for making a diagnosis of nongonococcal urethritis (NGU). Laboratory tests such as CBC, electrolytes, chest x-ray, and urine culture are not indicated. One could not argue with a blood cholesterol as part of caring for the overall health of an individual. In the next few years, screening for cholesterol levels will be as common as taking blood pressure. Urinalysis is not likely to be helpful in view of the urethral discharge. Scraping of the penile lesion is unnecessary. In view of his high risk behaviors, especially passive anal intercourse without a condom, a human immunodeficiency virus (HIV) antibody test should be done.

Further management at this time is to look at the gram stain for the presence of gram-negative intracellular diplococci. One could not argue with doing an RPR test for syphilis, but it will not help with immediate management, and ideally we will treat the patient with a regimen that is effective against incubating syphilis. The penile lesion is a venereal wart, and no further tests are necessary. It need not be confirmed by biopsy, and there are no lesions suggestive of syphilis (darkfield not indicated) or herpes (Tzanck prep not needed). We have a clear diagnosis of GC urethritis. Because of frequent co-existence of chlamydia, GC is now double treated with a regimen effective against both. If he were not at risk rectally, the treatment would be ampicillin 3.5g PO plus probenecid 1g PO, now, followed by tetracycline 500mg qid for one week. Because of the potential of rectal GC, he should be treated with a regimen effective for that (hence #41 is correct). Podophyllin should be applied to the wart. Small warts may respond to one treatment. If there is no effect after four weekly treatments, referral for Rx with liquid nitrogen is indicated. Certain strains of papillomavirus have been implicated as causative agents of cervical carcinoma. With increasing numbers of GC resistance nationwide, a follow-up test of cure should be arranged. Sexual partners need to be informed, evaluated, and epi treated. Safer sex counseling is highly appropriate, and if you have a ready supply of condoms in the office that reduces one more barrier (having to buy them) to their use.

Follow-up management in this case is critical. Most centers that do HIV antibody testing will actually perform three tests before calling the result positive. These include an ELISA test which is positive, a repeat ELISA test which is also positive, and a confirmatory more sensitive WESTERN BLOT test which is also positive. We are thus faced with a young, healthy, sexually active, adolescent, bisexual who is HIV antibody positive. As of August 1988, there were 70,000 cases of AIDS reported to the Centers for Disease Control. Many of these cases are in people in their twenties, which means they probably had initial contact with the virus in their teens. AIDS is the end-stage disease of infection with HIV. The Walter Reed staging system (Table 3.3) is an effective way to emphasize that infection with this virus is a continuum. What

TABLE 3.3. Walter Reed Staging System for Infection with HIV

Stage	WR-0	WR-1	WR-2	WR-3	WR-4	WR-5	WR-6
HIV antibody or virus isolation	−	+	+	+	+	+	+
Chronic lymphadenopathy	−	−	+	±	±	±	±
T-helper cells/mm3	>400	>400	>400	<400	<400	<400	<400
Delay hypersensitivity	N	N	N	N	P	P/C	P/C
Thrush	−	−	−	−	−	+	±
Opportunistic infection	−	−	−	−	−	−	+

N = normal
P = partial cutaneous anergy (response is intact to only one of these antigens: tetanus, mumps, candida, trichophyton)
C = complete anergy to all four

causes progression from one stage to another is unknown, as is the time it may take for such progression. Best estimates are that 50% or more of infected individuals will develop full-blown AIDS within 5–10 years of becoming HIV-antibody positive. The management of this young man at this time includes a PPD (the increase in tuberculosis nationwide is in part due to HIV infection), and an RPR (syphilis may act differently in people who are HIV-antibody positive: there may be a more rapid progression of syphilis, and more intense follow-up is needed). Sexual partners need to be referred to determine their HIV-antibody status. This is especially true in bisexuals in order to prevent perinatal transmission. IgG has no place in management, and it is highly inappropriate to suggest that casual contacts need to be evaluated, as it is to speak of a uniformly poor prognosis at this time. Referral to an "AIDS specialist" may be appropriate if available, though initial management can certainly be done by most practicing physicians. One may want to enquire to see if there are any trials of AZT (3′-azido-3′-deoxythymidine) in asymptomatic, HIV-antibody-positive individuals in your area. Review of what the patient needs to be alert to (lymphadenopathy, fatigue, fevers, weight loss, oral candidiasis) is appropriate, as is a discussion of how to prevent further transmission, including safer sex practices; avoiding donation of blood, sperm, or body organs; not sharing toothbrushes, razors, or other items that might be contaminated by blood; and cleaning surfaces contaminated with blood with household bleach (1 : 10 dilution with water). Many communities have developed programs for the "worried well," and referral to such an agency may be helpful.

Patient K

Scoring

K-1	K-2	K-3	K-4	K-5
1. +	11. +	20. 0	32. −	40. −
2. +	12. +	21. +	33. −	41. −
3. +	13. +	22. 0	34. 0	42. +
4. +	14. +	23. −	35. +	43. +
5. +	15. +	24. −	36. +	44. +
6. +	16. +	25. −	37. +	45. −
7. 0	17. 0	26. +	38. +	46. 0
8. 0	18. −	27. 0	39. −	
9. −	19. +	28. −		
10. +		29. −		
		30. −		
		31. +		

Discussion

The case presented is that of an infant who is having some difficulty with breastfeeding and is failing to thrive. The history is the most important element in this case, and it guides you to proper management. Course of the pregnancy, birth, and newborn period are all important points to explore carefully in the history. Previous problems and medical advice sought are also important to place the problem in perspective. We thus learn that the infant had a benign birth, then had some problems with jaundice, and was taken to see a physician who gave advice about sore nipples. At that time the infant had not yet regained her birth weight. This can be normal. Term babies can lose up to 10% of their birth weight, which they usually regain by a week, and by 10 days they are starting to gain weight. There should have been some follow-up of the case, both in terms of the jaundice and the mother's sore nipples. Had that occurred, the present state of affairs might have been avoided. Health of siblings and occupation of the father are noncontributory here but might have been helpful in terms of assessing what stresses the mother may be experiencing at home. To bring up a suggestion of retardation at this point would be a grave error, and one that would likely alienate and upset the parents for no good reason.

Physical exam is basically normal: liver edge palpable, knee clicks, open posterior fontanelle (closes by 6 to 8 weeks but may be closed at birth), and positive Babinski's sign are all common findings at this age, as is the lack of a social smile (begins around 6 weeks). Vaginal exam with a nasal speculum is not indicated. The presence of jaundice may be of concern and requires further investigation. A simian crease on one palm is considered a normal variant and may be present in up to 2% of normal children.

At this time, the only relevant lab studies are urinalysis (underlying urinary pathology can cause failure to thrive), bilirubin studies, and growth plotting. One could not argue with liver studies, CBC, and urine culture. To order the other studies is to proceed with expensive lab work before an adequate history has been taken. From the lab data, we learn that the indirect bilirubin is elevated and the direct is normal, thus confirming breastfeeding jaundice as one diagnosis (Table 3.4). The baby is dropping percentiles on the growth curve (see Figure 3.27).

TABLE 3.4. Breast Milk Jaundice

1. Does not alter the normal patterns of physiological jaundice. Jaundice in the first 4 days of life should not be considered to be breast milk jaundice.
2. Breast milk jaundice does not result in elevated levels of conjugated (direct) bilirubin.
3. The infant with breast milk jaundice appears well. Other causes of prolonged or late onset hyperbilirubinemia should be ruled out by history, physical examination, and simple laboratory data, including hematocrit, retic count, cord blood type, and Coombs' fractionation of bilirubin. Birth injury with hematoma, polycythemia, dehydration, infection, hemolytic process, hypothyroidism, intestinal obstruction, and liver disease are important causes to be ruled out.
4. The normal course of "untreated" breast milk jaundice is for levels to peak in the second or third week, with a gradual fall off by 6 to 8 weeks of life.
5. Interruption of breastfeeding may be indicated when the level approaches 20 mg% in a healthy, full-term infant.
6. Interruption of breastfeeding for 1 to 3 days results in a rapid decline in the level to about one half or less of the original value. This may be used as a diagnostic test.
7. Photototherapy has no place in the "treatment" of breast milk jaundice. It is an apparently benign, self-limited condition whose main importance lies in differentiating it from other, more serious conditions.

Excerpted from LaCerva, V: *Breastfeeding: A Manual for Health Professionals.* New York, Medical Examination Publishing Company, 1981.

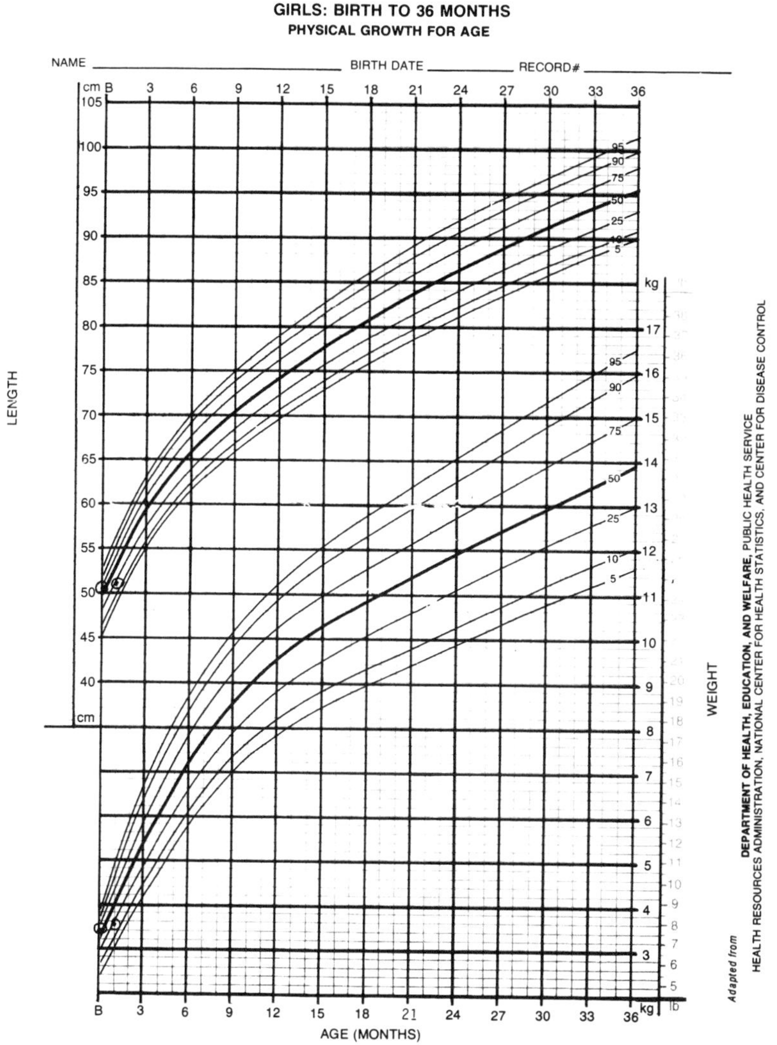

Figure 3.27

We have thus far ruled out the entire differential diagnosis of prolonged jaundice, which is lengthy and includes such unpleasant diagnoses as biliary atresia and neonatal hepatitis. We must now turn our attention to the lack of weight gain. The obvious place to start is with a more detailed feeding history. This leads us to learn that there are a number of breastfeeding problems. Mother has been using a nipple shield, which is a device that should never be recommended. It can interfere with the proper stimulation of the areolar tissue that stimulates the development of milk production if worn too long or too often during feedings. There are other, more effective ways to deal with sore nipples: change the baby's position; nurse from the least sore breast first; have more frequent, shorter feedings; apply a soothing cream (lanolin or even just olive oil); and avoid use of soaps or alcohol on the nipples. The point in the additional history that the nighttime feedings go easier suggests that mother may have some difficulty with let-down. This is confirmed by the infant's fussiness shortly after beginning a nursing. Fatigue, anxiety, stress, or poor support at home can all lead to decreased let-down. The third factor operative here is a lazy baby who is wanting to nurse only five times per day, instead of eight or more times. There is nothing to suggest that a sepsis work-up should be done at present or that a more extensive work-up for failure to thrive is indicated.

Proper management consists of adequate counseling and good follow-up. If the points mentioned above are remedied, this dyad can experience successfully breastfeeding. An actual prescription to stay in bed and nurse is a good start, as is discarding the nipple shield and offering the breast frequently to the infant. In this particular case, the infant was back on its normal growth curve within 3 weeks. Local support from the La Leche League and weekly encouraging visits to the doctor contributed to a successful outcome.

Patient L

Scoring

L-1	L-2	L-3	L-4	L-5	L-6
1. −	5. 0	12. 0	18. 0	23. 0	28. 0
2. 0	6. 0	13. 0	19. 0	24. 0	29. −
3. −	7. 0	14. 0	20. −	25. −	30. −
4. +	8. 0	15. 0	21. −	26. +	31. −
	9. 0	16. +	22. −	27. −	
	10. 0	17. −			
	11. −				

L-7	L-8	L-9	L-10	L-11	L-12
32. 0	35. 0	39. 0	43. 0	47. 0	50. −
33. −	36. 0	40. −	44. −	48. −	51. −
34. −	37. −	41. −	45. −	49. −	52. −
	38. −	42. −	46. 0		53. 0

Discussion

This 22-year-old man was well until about a month prior to coming to the emergency room. Without any known precipitant, he began to withdraw and became increasingly suspicious. When he was first seen, he showed looseness of associations and inappropriate affect. He complained of auditory hallucinations, thought insertion, thought broadcasting, and that the devil was trying to change him into a girl.

It is clear that this young man is suffering from an acute psychotic disorder. History and a drug screen rule out drug abuse. The physical examination rules out most other organic causes. His symptoms fit with the DSM-III-R criteria for a diagnosis of a schizophrenic-type disorder.

DSM-III-R diagnostic criteria separate into several subgroups: (1) a diagnosis of brief reactive psychosis is made when there is a strong psychosocial precipitant, and the disorder lasts more than a few hours but less than 1 month; (2) a diagnosis of schizophreniform disorder is made when the patient has symptoms that last more than 1 month but less than 6 months; (3) a diagnosis of schizophrenic disorder is made when the patient shows a deterioration from his previous levels of functioning in such areas as work, social relationships, and self-care over a period of 6 months or longer; (4) a diagnosis of psychotic disorder not otherwise specified is made when the patient does not meet the specific diagnostic criteria for other disorders or when not enough information is available to make a firm diagnosis.

From the information available, this young man is best categorized as having a schizophreniform disorder. He has been ill longer than 1 month but less than 6 months. Should he continue to show social and occupational decline, despite treatment, the diagnosis will be changed at the end of 6 months to that of schizophrenic disorder.

In the DSM-III-R diagnostic system, there are specific diagnostic criteria that must be met, critical time periods, and exclusion criteria. In the case of the schizophrenic-type disorders, the exclusion criteria rule out affective disorders and organicity.

In the past, we probably misdiagnosed many manics as schizophrenic. A strong affective component, a family history of mania or depression, previous manic or depressive episodes, and interpersonal intrusiveness should alert the clinician to the possibility of bipolar disorder. In this time of widespread drug abuse, it is also very important to rule out street drugs as well as prescribed drugs such as steroids. Although a fluctuating level of consciousness, disorientation (especially in time), poor recent memory, and visual hallucinations are the traditional hallmarks of organicity on the mental-status examination, some conditions, such as chronic amphetamine abuse and alcohol hallucinosis, are characterized by auditory hallucinations in a clear state of consciousness. Drug intoxication, withdrawal, hallucinosis, and delirium are all possibilities.

Phencyclidine (PCP or "angel dust") is now a common cause of psychotic drug-related emergency hospitalizations. It is characterized by nystagmus, elevated blood pressure, and muscular rigidity in an agitated, psychotic, or comatose patient whose respiration is not depressed. For these patients, major tranquilizers are contraindicated. The patient should be treated with partial sensory isolation in a darkened, quiet room and a minor tranquilizer, gastric lavage, and ammonium chloride (0.5 – 1 g po or nasogastric tube/6 h). For serious hypertension, diazoxide is useful.

Cannabis intoxication can lead to panic and transient paranoid reactions, as may have happened to this young man in the past.

DSM-III-R diagnostic criteria are very specific. Auditory hallucinations can be counted as evidence for a schizophrenic disorder, for example, only if they have certain characteristics, such as voices arguing or a voice giving a running commentary. Similarly, a delusion can be counted only if it is bizarre (eg, thought broadcasting) or is accompanied by prominent hallucination, incoherence, catatonic behavior, or flat or grossly inappropriate affect. This latter provision distinguishes the schizophrenic-type disorders from the paranoid disorders.

For the schizophrenic-type disorders, a major tranquilizer is indicated. With the exception of Sparine, they are all equally effective, given in equivalent doses, but they do differ in side effects and price. Rapid tranquilization is the treatment of choice for this young man. He was given haloperidol (Haldol) 5 mg po/hr until he became calm, then was given 5 mg bid and hs. The amount he needed was then titrated to his response.

All antipsychotic agents block dopamine receptors. However, one should not conclude that the psychosis is due to dopamine excess, a conclusion similar to conceptualizing pneumonia as an antibiotic-deficiency disease. Haloperidol was chosen because it seems the purest dopamine blocker, but any one of the antipsychotics might have been used.

All these drugs have side effects. For the high-potency group, basal ganglia side effects are particularly common: dystonia, akinesia, akathisia, parkinsonian syndrome, and tardive dyskinesia. Of these, tardive dyskinesia is the most serious and is frequently not reversible. Akathisia, the need to move about continuously, is the most common and may be confused with agitation.

This patient developed an acute dystonia affecting his sternocleidomastoid muscle. Dystonia is painful and frightening, but it responds to a wide variety of agents, anthihistamines such as Benadryl, caffeine, barbiturates, and antiparkinsonian agents. He was given one of the latter, Cogentin IM, and responded promptly.

Anticholinergic agents, such as Cogentin and Artane, can in themselves produce a delirium, as well as produce such problems as dry mouth, constipation, blurring of vision, exacerbation of acute-angle glaucoma, and urinary retention.

In addition to medication, the patient received supportive psychotherapy. He was discharged from the hospital after 6 days, and then treated in outpatient therapy for 6 months. Particular attention was paid to his social-support group because it has been found that a person's social network protects him against the effects of stressors and that, for schizophrenics, the social network often deteriorates remarkably after the first hospitalization. He did well, and a 2-year follow-up revealed he had graduated from college, married, and been continually employed.

Enlarged ventricles have been correlated with the so-called negative symptoms of schizophrenia: apathy, anergia, poverty of ideation, and flat affect. However, enlarged ventricles are not diagnostic. It would be clinically inappropriate to order a CT scan before doing a good history and physical examination. In this era of cost consciousness, it would also be administratively intolerable.

There are several distractors dealing with depression among these questions. Although it now can no longer be accepted fully, it has been useful to consider severe depressions as related to functional synaptic deficits in either serotonin (5-hydroxy-tryptamine) or norepinephrine. Found in the urine, 3,4-MHPG is a breakdown product and is believed to reflect levels of synaptic norepinephrine in the brain. Found in the cerebrospinal fluid, 5-HIAA is the comparable breakdown product for serotonin. There is no reason to order these expensive tests in this case.

The DST has been useful in determining when antidepressant medication may be useful in the treatment of depression and when, after the patient has recovered, it is possible to discontinue it. The test is based on the fact that when dexamethasone is given, normal people show a consequent suppression of cortisol. Some depressed people do not. These are patients with endogenous depression (DSM-III-R symptoms of melancholia). The lack of suppression is believed to reflect hypothalamic-pituitary-adrenal axis dysfunction. It is this group of nonsuppressors who are most likely to respond positively to antidepressants. Unfortunately, this test is not as specific as we had once hoped. People with other psychiatric disorders, such as Alzheimer's disease and mania, as well as major infections, febrile diseases, cardiac or pulmonary diseases, or who have had surgery, frequently demonstrate nonsuppression. However, it has spurred interest in seeking other biological markers for depression. There is no reason to order it for this patient.

References

1. American Psychiatric Association. *Diagnostic and Statistical Manual of Mental Disorders*, ed 3, revised. Washington, DC, American Psychiatric Association Press, 1987, pp 187–199.

2. Allen JR, Allen BA: *Psychiatry: A Guide*. Garden City, NY, Medical Examination Publishing Company, 1983.

3. Kaplan HI, Sadock BJ: *Modern Synopsis of Comprehensive Textbook of Psychiatry*. Baltimore, Williams and Wilkins, 1985, pp 194–255.

4. Winokur G, Clayton P: *The Medical Basis of Psychiatry*. Philadelphia, WB Saunders, 1986, pp 80–115.

Patient M

Scoring

M-1	M-2	M-3	M-4	M-5	M-6
1. +	8. 0	15. +	22. −	27. −	32. +
2. +	9. +	16. +	23. +	28. 0	33. +
3. −	10. +	17. +	24. +	29. +	34. −
4. +	11. +	18. +	25. −	30. −	35. −
5. +	12. −	19. −	26. 0	31. +	36. 0
6. +	13. +	20. −			37. −
7. 0	14. −	21. +			38. −

Discussion

This middle-aged white man presented with a fairly typical history of jaundice and upper abdominal pain of short duration. The important point in the history was that he had a previous operation. Jaundiced patients do not feel like eating fatty foods and in general their appetite is poor. He also gave a history of fever, which in the presence of jaundice and pain should raise the possibility of cholangitis. The loss of appetite and the fever should also raise the possibility of hepatitis; one should look for a cause. On further evaluation, it was apparent that the patient had a previous operation, at which time he sustained an injury to the common bile duct. The most common cause of common bile duct injury is a surgical procedure. Cholecystectomy is the most common operation and distal gastrectomy or antrectomy is the second most common operation resulting in this injury. The patient had undergone a choledochoduodenostomy at the time for management of his common duct injury. It is important to get the history of blood transfusions, but most cases of hepatitis due to blood transfusion present within 3 months of the event. One should inquire about the patient's use of different drugs and alcohol as possible causes of the jaundice.

In clinical evaluation, it was apparent that the patient had a previous operation and he had a scar. Evaluation should be carried out for any abdominal mass. In middle-aged individuals the most common causes of surgical jaundice are either cancer of the head of the pancreas or common bile duct stones. In the presence of cancer of the pancreas, one might see ascites. This also may be seen in patients with cirrhosis and associated jaundice. Rash and scratch marks on the skin indicate extrahepatic biliary obstruction and cholangitis. Murphy's sign is not seen in the absence of the gallbladder and is only of value in the diagnosis of acute cholecystitis. Physical examination should include a rectal examination to check for a rectal cancer or a Blumer's shelf due to other abdominal malignancies. At the conclusion of the rectal examination, one should check for blood in the stool by a guaiac test. Cancers of the ampulla of Vater or of the duodenum could produce obstructive jaundice and also a positive stool guaiac. Caput medusae is a sign of advanced portal hypertension and is a dilatation of the periumbilical veins. In the absence of history of alcoholism and other evidence of cirrhosis, this finding is seldom seen.

The most important results are in the liver profile (see Table 3.1). This shows that the patient has a fairly significant jaundice with a serum bilirubin of 9.2 mg% and, additionally, he has a significant elevation of serum alkaline phosphatase. The latter is particularly indicative of obstructive jaundice. Although the SGOT and LDH are elevated, these elevations are mild and are consistent with obstructive jaundice. When jaundice is due to hepatocellular causes, these enzyme values are significantly elevated. The hemogram indicates a normal hemoglobin and hematocrit. Serum electrolytes were also normal and one should check the gross renal function in patients with jaundice. The serum protein values indicate a fairly good state of nutrition. In an otherwise healthy individual, arterial blood gases are not routinely performed. The urine urobilinogen is a very useful and simple test. In complete obstructive jaundice the urine would be negative for urobilinogen. This test is underutilized but is very helpful. In patients with jaundice one should check prothrombin time and, if abnormal, this should be corrected prior to any operative procedures.

In the radiologic evaluation of jaundiced patients, the most useful exams are ultrasonography and a transhepatic cholangiogram. In the presence of jaundice of the level seen in this patient, the IV cholangiogram is a useless test. Ultrasonography, on the other hand, will indicate dilated ducts, and the presence of a mass in the head of the pancreas can also be appreciated by this study. If there are stones in the common duct, an ultrasonogram is useful in diagnosing the same. The superior mesenteric angiogram is performed when the diagnosis of cancer of the head of the pancreas is made or if there is a mass in the pancreas, the nature of which is not very clear. The procedure has been replaced by CT scanning and is no longer performed on a routine basis. An ERCP is also useful in the evaluation of jaundice; however, in this particular patient, who has a Billroth II anastomosis, the test is going to be extremely difficult because the endoscopist has to cannulate the afferent loop of the gastrojejunal anastomosis and identify the ampulla, or in this particular case identify the stricture at the site of the choledochoduodenal anastomosis. Except in the hands of some extremely competent people, this test is not of value in this particular patient. The transhepatic cholangiogram (see Figure 3.22) shows a choledochoduodenal anastomosis with a stricture. Proximal to the stricture, the common bile duct is dilated and shows radiolucent defects that are probably stones. The intrahepatic ducts are also dilated, indicating a fairly prolonged period of partial obstruction.

The patient needs surgical correction of this problem, but prior to his operation he should be adequately prepared. The most important step in this particular patient is to put him on parenteral antibiotics. This should be started prior to the transhepatic cholangiography because the procedure itself might introduce infection or result in dissemination of infected bile into the system. Drugs that are used in this situation are a combination of an aminoglycoside, such as gentamicin, and a cephalosporin, such as cefazolin. These two antibiotics together would cover most common biliary bacteria. At the time of the transhepatic cholangiogram, a sample of bile should be obtained for culture and sensitivity. At the conclusion of cholangiography, the radiologist should leave a catheter in the biliary system. This would decompress the biliary system and reduce the jaundice. It is known that there is a high risk of postoperative renal failure in patients who have been operated on for obstructive jaundice. Preoperative biliary drainage reduces this risk. The patient's hemoglobin and hematocrit were normal and his serum proteins were also normal. Therefore, preoperative blood transfusion is not indicated. On the other hand, he might have a stormy and prolonged postoperative course due to the fact that he is being operated on for a recurrent stricture and hyperalimentation could be begun a day or two prior to the operation. The patient does need vitamin K supplementation but this should be accomplished by parenteral routes. Oral vitamin supplementation, particularly of the fat-soluble vitamins, is useless in the presence of obstructive jaundice.

The operation of choice in this patient depends on the situation at the time of operation. The patient does have a fairly decent length of common bile duct. It is feasible in this situation to revise the anastomosis or reconstruct a new choledochoduodenostomy. If the duodenum is scarred because of previous surgery, one could consider performing a choledochojejunostomy. If the stump of the common bile duct is short, it then can be converted into hepaticojejunostomy, but as long as a decent length of the common duct is available this should be used to construct a choledochojejunostomy. Choledochogastrostomy is not desirable because the diversion of bile into the stomach will produce bile gastritis and discomfort. Additionally, this patient has no distal stomach and, therefore, the procedure is not feasible. Choledochotomy and removal of stones is not the answer to the problem because he is producing stones proximal to his stricture. The stricture should be surgically revised so that there is no stasis and thus prevent recurrence. The Longmire procedure is only performed when one cannot find a remnant of the common hepatic duct or any major duct at the porta hepatis. In those situations a left hepatic lobectomy and anastomosis of a Roux-en-Y loop of jejunum to the left hepatic duct may be required. In this patient, there was a good length of the common duct, and therefore it is not indicated. Endoscopic papillotomy in this patient is of no value, as noted earlier. The endoscope has to reach the second part of the duodenum through a gastrojejunal anastomosis. Further, the stricture was not in the papilla but was at the site of a previous choledochoduodenostomy.

Strictures of common bile ducts are very difficult problems. The most common cause of injury to the common bile duct is a previous surgical procedure such as a cholecystectomy or gastrectomy. Care should be exercised in performing these procedures. The initial repair should be performed meticulously in all cases. Recurrence of strictures do occur and contribute to recurrent cholangitis, obstructive jaundice, and even biliary cirrhosis.

References

1. Schwartz SI (ed): *Principles of Surgery,* ed 4. New York, McGraw-Hill, 1984, pp 1055–1059, 1320–1329, 1339–1340.

2. Sabiston DC (ed): *Textbook of Surgery*, ed 13. Philadelphia, WB Saunders, 1986, pp 1132–1134, 1154–1161.

Patient N

Scoring

N-1	N-2	N-3	N-4	N-5
1. +	10. +	16. +	23. 0	30. +
2. +	11. +	17. +	24. −	31. −
3. +	12. +	18. −	25. 0	32. −
4. +	13. −	19. −	26. +	33. 0
5. 0	14. +	20. −	27. +	34. +
6. +	15. +	21. +	28. 0	35. −
7. −		22. −	29. −	
8. +				
9. +				

Discussion

This 65-year-old obese white man was admitted with lower abdominal colicky pain of 3-days' duration. The location of the pain in the left lower quadrant and in the suprapubic area should raise a suspicion of an inflammatory lesion. The history of similar attacks of pain in the previous year might lead one to think of diverticulitis. This goes along with increasing constipation and episodes of diarrhea. However, the possibility that this may be due to a cancer should also be kept in mind. Either of these conditions could produce some degree of large bowel obstruction. However, this has not reached the point in this patient to make him vomit. He does have constipation and has not passed any gas. The admitting vital signs revealed an elevated temperature and this should further confirm the suspicion of an inflammatory bowel problem such as diverticulitis or a perforation due to a cancer.

Patients with diverticular disease do not often bleed. When bleeding occurs, it is usually the massive variety and generally stops spontaneously. On the other hand, patients with cancer of the colon might have no obvious bleeding but have steady blood loss. Conditions such as ulcerative colitis, however, are associated with bloody diarrhea. The increased use of laxatives should indicate a progressively narrowing lesion in the large bowel and this could be either an inflammatory stricture or a malignant process. The absence of weight loss reduces the possibility of malignancy.

The patient has urinary symptoms of the nature of dysuria and frequency. This is not unusual in this age group, at which time patients first present prostatic symptoms. In a patient with history suggestive of inflammatory process, one should think of the process extending to the bladder wall. In addition, an enlarged prostate could be responsible for the same. In this obese individual diagnosis of an abdominal mass is not easy. However, localized tenderness in the left lower quadrant is strongly suggestive of diverticulitis. Once the diverticulitis is localized, the bowel sounds may be normal. Only when there is a free perforation is the abdomen completely silent. A rectal examination is necessary and the stool should be checked for guaiac. In diverticulitis, it might localize the tenderness, and in the presence of a low-lying cancer this can be felt. The initial work-up revealed an elevated white cell count with left shift. This strongly supports the suspicion of an inflammatory process such as diverticulitis. Blood cultures were negative because this was a localized lesion. The urine culture showed predominantly fecal organisms and one should suspect an extension of the inflammatory process into the bladder. Stool cultures are of no value in this patient. Plain abdominal series are useful in determining the gas pattern and evidence of bowel obstruction. When there is a free perforation due to diverticulitis, the x-ray film will show free air in the abdomen. A useful procedure at this stage is ultrasonography. In this patient, this revealed a mass. Sometimes the sonogram might reveal the presence of an abscess and indicate the need for early exploration and drainage.

The initial management of diverticulitis is by conservative measures. The patient should be on IV fluids and, if necessary, nasogastric suction. Parenteral antibiotics, including gentamicin and either clindamycin or metronidazole, would be useful in controlling local infection. In acute diverticulitis the patient would not have any oral intake, and oral neomycin and erythromycin have no value. Similarly, bulk laxatives are only useful in the conservative management of diverticular disease but have no role in the management of acute diverticulitis. A cecostomy is not useful. Most patients are treated conservatively, and if they do not resolve or develop one of the complications, then surgery would be considered. A proximal colostomy alone, even in the presence of perforated diverticulitis, is not as useful as a colostomy combined with drainage of the involved segment or resection.

In the presence of diverticulitis, sigmoidoscopy is often not helpful. The scope can seldom advance past the sigmoid flexure due to spasm and even then it may only show some pus or mucus trickling down. A CT scan is an unnecessary and costly procedure. The patient, as noted in the history and management, has passed air or gas along with urine. This should raise a strong suspicion of colovesical fistula. The most useful methods for diagnosing this are a cystogram and cystoscopy. The cystogram presented in Figure 3.23 shows a fistula and appearance of the contrast in a bowel loop. Urethrogram is only indicated when feces or air are leaking through the meatus irrespective of bladder contraction or attempts at micturition. A colonoscopy does not help in pointing to the site of fistula but only confirms the presence of an inflammatory area, normal or inflamed mucosa, and perhaps a diagnosis of diverticular disease.

The ideal treatment of a patient with colovesical fistula due to diverticular disease is primary resection of the involved segment of colon, repair of the site of fistula in the bladder, and suprapubic drainage. The continuity of the bowel is to be reestablished by primary anastomosis through healthy areas. When there is severe inflammation or an abscess formation at the site of the fistula, one might elect to do a sigmoid resection, proximal colostomy and bladder repair with drainage, and subsequently closing of the colostomy. In the management of colovesical fistula of this nature, hyperalimentation and bladder drainage alone have no value. These fistulae do not heal because of constant infection from the fecal stream. Similarly, proximal colostomy alone is of no value. It might divert the fecal stream, but the feces in the bowel distal to the colostomy will continue to infect the bladder, and further, the fistula will not heal. The patient does not have evidence of hypertrophic prostate, and therefore transurethral prostatectomy has no value in this situation.

References

1. Schwartz SI (ed): *Principles of Surgery,* ed 4. New York, McGraw-Hill, 1984, pp 1187–1190.

2. Sabiston DC (ed): *Textbook of Surgery,* ed 13. Philadelphia, WB Saunders, 1986, pp 997–999.

Patient O

Scoring

O-1	O-2	O-3	O-4	O-5	O-6
1. +	7. +	13. +	24. −	36. −	43. +
2. +	8. +	14. +	25. 0	37. +	44. +
3. 0	9. +	15. −	26. +	38. −	45. +
4. +	10. +	16. +	27. +	39. 0	46. 0
5. +	11. +	17. 0	28. −	40. +	47. −
6. +	12. +	18. −	29. −	41. −	48. −
		19. +	30. −	42. −	49. +
		20. −	31. +		50. −
		21. +	32. +		
		22. +	33. +		
		23. +	34. +		
			35. −		

Discussion

The presentation of this 70-year-old man with increasing constipation, weakness, dark stools, and fatigue should lead to a strong suspicion of cancer of the left colon. The patient does have a long history of constipation, but the important feature is the change in the bowel habits in the recent past. The episodes of diarrhea are probably related to fecal impaction and consequent mucus secretion. The weight loss also suggests a diagnosis of malignancy of the colon.

It is interesting to note that the patient did have a barium enema performed 4 years prior to this admission, at which time he was found to have diverticular disease. It is also of interest that he had a previous aortoiliac bypass for aortic aneurysm. At that time, as in most instances, perhaps his inferior mesenteric artery was tied off. The surgeon at that time would have examined the colon and excluded a possible cancer at that stage. The family history is useful to make sure that there are no other contributory factors but is not valuable in diagnosis. Most patients with a history of familial polyposis develop their cancer at a very early age, and so it is unlikely that is a contributing factor in this man. The nature of bleeding with colonic cancer is such to produce melena. On the other hand, massive colorectal bleeding is seen in diverticular disease. Although the patient is known to have diverticular disease, the nature of his bleeding does not indicate that it is due to the same. The increasing usage of laxatives indicates that his colonic lumen was perhaps being compromised, and he was developing some degree of intestinal obstruction. Older individuals take a large number of medicines and it is important to check if the patient is on any medicines that are likely to produce bleeding (eg, potassium supplements, antiarthritic medications).

Patients with left colon strictures may have abdominal distention due to partial intestinal obstruction. This patient has undergone an aortoiliac anastomosis in the past and may have had a segment of ischemic colitis. Therefore, in addition to strictures due to diverticular disease and malignancy, one should consider ischemic colitis as a cause. Left colon lesions are seldom palpable as a mass, although a mass may be palpable in a number of patients with right colon cancer. Once a suspicion of colonic cancer is entertained, one should evaluate the patient for extent of the disease in terms of liver metastases and ascites. This patient did not demonstrate these findings. Rectal examination and examination of the stool for guaiac is an absolute necessity in any patient with these symptoms. In this patient, the lesion is too far above (30 cm from the anus) to be felt with examining finger, but the stool was positive for guaiac, indicating some bleeding.

The initial investigations include the standard ones for any surgical patient; however, it should be noted that this patient's serum electrolytes show a significant hyponatremia, hypokalemia, and hypochloremia. In patients with a colonic lesion, such as electrolyte abnormality, a suspicion of a villous adenoma should be raised. The fact that this patient had diarrhea, off and on, should increase the suspicion. The hemogram shows that the patient is anemic; this could be due partly to actual blood loss and partly to a dilutional effect. Serum amylase was not indicated in this patient because acute pancreatic disease was not suspected. The liver profile is a useful investigation not only to determine liver function but also to evaluate for any evidence of metastatic disease (indicated by abnormal liver enzymes, hyperbilirubinemia, etc.). A chest x-ray is a requirement in any elderly patient who is likely to be operated on to evaluate his lungs and heart and also to serve as a baseline in case the patient develops a lung lesion at a later time. It should, however, be remembered that pulmonary metastases are very uncommon with colonic cancer. A plain abdominal series in this patient is useless. Most radiologists obtain a plain film of the abdomen prior to doing an upper GI series or a barium enema. Therefore, as a separate study it has no value. A sigmoidoscopy is absolutely indicated; however, in this patient the lesion was more proximal and was not useful. An OCG was not indicated since biliary disease was not being seriously considered. An upper GI series is useful in evaluation because the patient does have bleeding per rectum. This study would exclude proximal causes of melena, such as cancer of the stomach, bleeding varices, or a duodenal ulcer. Occasionally, small bowel polyps account for the melena. Colon cancers may produce blockage of the ureters, particularly on the left side, and, therefore, an IVP is indicated. It is preferable to do this on the same day as doing the barium enema but prior to the enema because once the barium is introduced to the colon, it may cause problems in interpretation of the IVP. The most useful of these tests is the barium enema; this shows the constricting lesion (see Figure 3.24) in the sigmoid bowel. The barium enema also indicates the coexistent diverticular disease. The picture is not consistent with a stricture due to ischemic colitis and, in fact, has a fairly typical "apple-core" appearance. However, in view of the fact that the patient did have diverticular disease, one has to differentiate the stricture of diverticulitis from that due to malignant disease.

The further studies are to determine the cause of the stricture more precisely and to plan the management. An upper endoscopy and biopsy are, therefore, not indicated on the basis of the previous studies. Colonoscopy and biopsy are also not indicated for a lesion at this level. In further management, the patient should have a replacement of electrolytes to correct the abnormalities. In addition, a serum CEA level should be obtained as a baseline because it would prove useful in subsequent management. It also is helpful in the diagnosis of cancer of the colon. Urinary 5-HIAA levels are not indicative because there is no evidence of carcinoid syndrome or of carcinoid tumor. Serum alpha-fetoprotein levels are useful in the evaluation of hepatic tumors, not colon cancers. Mesenteric angiography is not indicated in this patient. The degree of bleeding is a slow, steady one and is not significantly brisk to be useful in localization of the bleeding site. Further, in this patient at the time of the aneurysm, the inferior mesenteric artery was probably ligated, and, therefore, there was no indication for it. The patient is anemic; preoperatively, he should be transfused so that he can tolerate anesthesia. Similarly, he should be started on parenteral hyperalimentation because of his previous weight loss and age and because he was probably nutritionally depleted. There is no need for parenteral vitamin K because the patient has no evidence of any obstructive jaundice. At this stage, consideration should be given to elective resection of the colonic lesion and the bowel should be prepared. Bowel preparation includes mechanical bowel preparation, both from below and also by using liquid diets and laxatives orally. In addition to mechanical bowel preparation, the patient should be given oral nonabsorbable antibiotics such as neomycin and erythromycin-base preparations to reduce the bacterial flora and the infective complications of bowel resection.

The ideal procedure for treatment of the lesions shown is a primary resection including a good length of bowel proximally and distally. Such length should include at least 10 cm on each side, and a primary anastomosis can be performed. However, if at the time of resection there were other factors such as tension at the anastomosis or risk of leakage, one could do a resection of the tumor and a proximal colostomy with the idea of going back into the abdomen for a second-stage closure of the colostomy. That is an acceptable alternative. Since the patient does not have any acute emergency such as an obstruction, the three-stage procedure is not recommended. In the past, when antibiotics were not available or the patient was an emergency, a three-stage procedure was often considered. Abdominoperineal resection is not indicated because even by removing 10 cm distally, the patient would still have decent length of rectum and an anastomosis can be performed. Bulk laxatives, antispasmodics, and other conservative measures are useful in the management of diverticular disease, and they are not of value when the patient has a stricture. Similarly, local excision or fulguration is inadequate. Fulguration by itself might result in perforation of the colon in this lesion and sepsis and death.

Presuming that the patient has had no metastatic disease in the liver or in the peritoneal cavity and has undergone a primary resection with anastomosis, he should be carefully followed periodically for evidence of recurrence. Sigmoidoscopy is simple and should be performed at quarterly intervals. The anastomosis itself probably would be in the reach of the sigmoidoscopy and the area should be examined for any suture line or other recurrence. Since the patient has had colon cancer, he should be examined colonoscopically annually and barium enema is an acceptable alternative. A chest x-ray is not a high priority since colon cancer most often spreads to the liver and it is only in the late stages that there are any lung lesions. There is no value in doing serum alpha-fetoprotein levels or urinary 5-HIAA levels in this patient. On the other hand, if after the operation, the patient's serum CEA levels were within the normal range and subsequently they were elevated, it would indicate a recurrence or metastatic disease. Therefore, CEA levels should be measured. Quarterly CT scans of the abdomen are not justified. When one is looking for metastatic disease in the liver, ultrasonography or a liver function test would be equally useful. A CT scan is only indicated if there is some suspicion of metastatic disease based on other tests. A routine CT scan is economically unjustified.

This patient is an interesting problem because he has a colonic lesion that could have been due to diverticulitis, ischemic colitis, or cancer. In the postoperative management, the value of sigmoidoscopy and CEA levels cannot be overemphasized.

References

1. Schwartz EI (ed): *Principles of Surgery,* ed 4. New York, McGraw-Hill, 1984, pp 1050–1051, 1192–1193, 1197–1210.

2. Sabiston DC (ed): *Textbook of Surgery,* ed 13. Philadelphia, WB Saunders, 1986, pp 988–990, 1003–1009.

PATIENT MANAGEMENT PROBLEMS: RESPONSES

Responses

For each course of action chosen, there are corresponding responses in this section. Use the enclosed special pen to reveal the concealed information. Apply the pen LIGHTLY from left to right after the number of the response to visualize the response (which ends at the asterisk*) corresponding to the course(s) of action chosen.

Sample Responses (Visualize All 3)

1. Use the pen LIGHTLY*
2. Only until the asterisk is visualized*
3. Now begin*

Patient A

A-1. 1.

2.

3.

4.

5.

6.

A-2. 7.

8.

9.

10.

11.

12.

A-3. 13.

14.

15.

16.

17.

18.

A-4. 19.

20.

21.

22.

23.

24.

A-5. 25.

26.

27.

28.

29.

30.

A-6. 31.

32.

33. [illegible]

34.

35. [illegible]

36.

A-7. 37. [illegible]

38.

39.

40.

41.

42.

43. [illegible]

A-8. 44. [illegible]

45.

46.

47.

48.

49.

A-9. 50.

51.

52.

53.

54.

55.

A-10. 56.

57.

58.

59.

60.

61.

END OF RESPONSES FOR PATIENT A

Patient B

B-1. 1.

2.

3.

4.

5.

6.

B-2. 7. [illegible]

8.

9.

10. [illegible]

11. [illegible]

12. [illegible]

13. [illegible]

B-3. 14. [illegible]

15.

16.

17. [illegible]

18. [illegible]

19. [illegible]

20.

B-4. 21.

22.

23. [illegible]

24.

25.

26.

27.

B-5. 28.

29.

30.

31.

32.

33.

B-6. 34.

35.

36.

37.

38.

39.

40.

END OF RESPONSES FOR PATIENT B

Patient C

C-1. 1.

2.

3.

4.

5.

6.

7.

C-2.

8.

9.

10.

11.

12.

C-3. 13.

14.

15.

16.

17.

18.

19. [illegible]

SMA 12		Normal value
SGOT	140	(7–40)
LDH (lactate dehydrogenase)	255	(100–225)
Alkaline phosphatase	125	(30–1[illegible]5)
Total bilirubin	2.0	(0.2–1.2)
Creatinine	0.8	(0.7–1.4)
Uric acid	3	(2.2–7.7)
Glucose	95	(65–110)
Cholesterol	10[illegible]	([illegible]–240)
Inorganic phosphorus	4	(2.[illegible]–[illegible].5)
Calcium	9	(8.[illegible]–10.[illegible])
Albumin	4	(3.[illegible]–5.2)
Total protein	7	(6.[illegible]–[illegible].5)

C-4. 20. [illegible]

21. [illegible]

22. [illegible]

23.

24.

C-5. 25.

26. [illegible]

	2	3	4	5	6	8	[illegible]				
	1200	150	[illegible]	400	600	500	275	[illegible]	[illegible]	[illegible]	40
Bilirubin	[illegible]	2.8	[illegible]	[illegible]	[illegible]	[illegible]	4.0	[illegible]	[illegible]	[illegible]	2.6
[illegible]	[illegible]	[illegible]	[illegible]	[illegible]	[illegible]	[illegible]	[illegible]	[illegible]	[illegible]	[illegible]	[illegible]

27. [illegible]

28.

C-6. 29.

30. [illegible] showed evidence of piecemeal necrosis and bridging but without evidence of cirrhosis.

31. [illegible]

32.

END OF RESPONSES FOR PATIENT C

Patient D

D-1. 1. [illegible]

2.

3.

4. [illegible]

D-2. 5.

6. [illegible]

7. [illegible]

8.

9. [illegible]

10.

D-3. 11. [illegible]

12. [illegible]

13. [illegible]

14.

15.

16.

17.

18.

D-4. 19.

20.

21.

22.

23.

24.

D-5. 25.

26.

27.

28.

29.

D-6. 30.

31.

32.

33.

34.

35.

D-7. 36.

37.

38.

39.

40.

D-8. 41.

42.

43.

D-9. 44.

45.

46.

47.

48.

49.

50.

51.

52.

53.

54.

55.

56.

57.

58.

59.

60.

D-10. 61.

62.

D-11. 63.

64.

65.

66.

67.

68.

69.

70.

D-12. 71.

72.

73.

74.

75.

76.

77.

78.

END OF RESPONSES FOR PATIENT D

Patient E

E-1. 1.

2.

3.

4.

5.

E-2. 6.

7.

8.

9.

10.

11.

12.

E-3. 13.

14.

15.

16.

17.

18.

19.

20.

E-4. 21.

22.

23.

24.

25.

26.

27.

28.

29.

30.

31.

32.

33.

E-5. 34.

35.

36.

37.

38.

39.

E-6. 40.

41.

42.

43.

44.

45.

46.

E-7. 47.

48.

49.

50.

51.

52.

53.

54.

55.

E-8. 56.

57.

58.

59.

60.

61.

E-9. 62.

63.

64.

65.

66.

E-10. 67.

68.

69.

70.

END OF RESPONSES FOR PATIENT E

Patient F

F-1. 1.

2.

3.

4. [illegible]

5. [illegible]

6. [illegible]

7. [illegible]

8.

F-2. 9. [illegible]

10. [illegible]

11. [illegible]

12. [illegible]

13. [illegible]

14. [illegible]

15. [illegible]

F-3. 16.

17. [illegible]

18. [illegible]

19. [illegible]

20.

21. [illegible]

F-4. 22. [illegible]

23.

24. [illegible]

25.

26.

F-5. 27.

28.

29.

30.

31.

F-6. 32.

33.

34.

35.

36.

37.

END OF RESPONSES FOR PATIENT F

Patient G

G-1. 1.

2.

3.

4. [illegible]

5. [illegible]

6.

G-2. 7. [illegible]

8. [illegible]

9.

10.

11.

12.

G-3. 13. [illegible]

14.

15. [illegible]

16. [illegible]

17. [illegible]

18. [illegible]

G-4. 19. [illegible]

20. [illegible]

21.

22.

23.

24. [illegible]

G-5. 25.

26.

27.

28.

29.

30.

G-6. 31.

32.

33.

34.

35.

36.

END OF RESPONSES FOR PATIENT G

Patient H

H-1. 1.

2.

3.

4.

5.

6.

H-2. 7.

8.

9.

10.

11.

12.

13.

H-3. 14.

15.

16.

17.

18.

19.

H-4. 20.

21.

22.

23.

24.

25.

26.

27.

H-5. 28.

29. [illegible]

30.

31.

H-6. 32.

33.

34.

35. [illegible]

36.

37.

END OF RESPONSES FOR PATIENT H

Patient I

I-1. 1. [illegible]

2. [illegible]

3. [illegible]

4. [illegible]

5. [illegible]

6. [illegible]

7.

8. [illegible]

I-2. 9. [illegible]

10. [illegible]

11. [illegible]

12. [illegible]

13. [illegible]

14. [illegible]

15. [illegible]

16. [illegible]

I-3. 17. [illegible]

18. [illegible]

19.

20. [illegible]

21. [illegible]

22. [illegible]

23.

I-4. 24.

25.

26.

27.

28.

29.

30.

I-5. 31.

32.

33.

34.

I-6. 35.

36.

37.

38.

39.

END OF RESPONSES FOR PATIENT I

Patient J

J-1. 1. [illegible]

2. [illegible]

3. [illegible]

4. [illegible]

5.

6. [illegible]

7. [illegible]

8. [illegible]

9. [illegible]

10. [illegible]

11. [illegible]

12.

J-2. 13. [illegible]

14.

15.

16. [illegible]

17. [illegible]

18. [illegible]

19. [illegible]
[illegible]

20. [illegible]

J-3. 21. [illegible]

22. [illegible]

23.

24. [illegible]

25. [illegible]
[illegible]

26. [illegible]

27. [illegible]

28. [illegible]

29. [illegible]

30. [illegible]

31. [illegible]

32. [illegible]

33.

J-4. 34.

35.

36.

37.

38.

39.

J-5. 40.

41.

42.

43.

44.

45.

46.

47.

J-6. 48.

49.

50.

51.

52.

53.

54.

55.

56.

57.

58.

END OF RESPONSES FOR PATIENT J

Patient K

K-1. 1.

2.

3.

4.

5.

6.

7.

8.

9.

10.

[illegible]

K-2. 11. [illegible]

12. [illegible]

13. [illegible]

14. [illegible]

15. [illegible]

16. [illegible]

17. [illegible]

18.

19.

K-3. 20. [illegible]

21.

22.

23.

24. [illegible]

25. [illegible]

26. [illegible]

27. [illegible]

28. [illegible]

29. [illegible]

30. [illegible]

31. [illegible]

K-4. 32.

33. [illegible]

34. [illegible]

35. [illegible]

36.

37. [illegible]

38. [illegible]

39.

K-5. 40.

41.

42.

43.

44.

45.

46.

END OF RESPONSES FOR PATIENT K

Patient L

L-1. 1.

2.

3.

4.

L-2. 5.

6.

7.

8.

9.

10.

11.

L-3. 12.

13.

14.

15.

16.

17.

L-4. 18.

19.

20.

21.

22.

L-5. 23.

24.

25.

26.

27.

L-6. 28.

29.

30.

31.

L-7. 32.

33.

34.

L-8. 35.

36.

37.

38.

L-9. 39.

40.

41.

42.

L-10. 43.

44.

45.

46.

L-11. 47.

48.

49.

L-12. 50.

51.

52.

53.

END OF RESPONSES FOR PATIENT L

Patient M

M-1. 1.

2.

3.

4.

5.

6.

7.

M-2. 8.

9.

10.

11.

12.

13.

14.

M-3. 15.

16.

17.

18.

19.

20.

21.

M-4. 22.

23.

24.

25.

26.

M-5. 27.

28. [illegible]

29.

30.

31. [illegible]

M-6. 32. [illegible]

33. [illegible]

34.

35.

36.

37.

38. [illegible]

END OF RESPONSES FOR PATIENT M

Patient N

N-1. 1. [illegible]

2.

3. [illegible]

4. [illegible]

5. [illegible]

6. [illegible]

7.

8. [illegible]

9. [illegible]

N-2. 10. [illegible]

11. [illegible]

12. [illegible]

13. [illegible]

14. [illegible]

15.

N-3. 16. [illegible]

17.

18.

19.

20.

21. [illegible]

22.

N-4. 23.

24.

25. [illegible]

26.

27. [illegible]

28. [illegible]

29.

N-5. 30.

31.

32.

33.

34. [illegible]

35.

END OF RESPONSES FOR PATIENT N

Patient O

O-1. 1. [illegible]

2. [illegible]

3.

4. [illegible]

5.

6. [illegible]

O-2. 7. [illegible]

8. [illegible]

9. [illegible]

10.

11. [illegible]

12. [illegible]

O-3. 13. [illegible]

14. [illegible]

15.

16. [illegible]

17. [illegible]

18.

19. [illegible]

20.

21.

22.

23. [illegible]

O-4. 24.

25. [illegible]

26. [illegible]

27. [illegible]

28.

29.

30.

31.

32.

33.

34.

35.

O-5. 36.

37.

38.

39.

40.

41.

42.

O-6. 43.

44.

45.

46.

47.

48.

49. [illegible]

50. [illegible]

END OF RESPONSES FOR PATIENT O